WOMEN SEX POWER& PLEASURE

ALSO BY EVELYN RESH

The Secret Lives of Teen Girls: What Your Mother Wouldn't Talk about but Your Daughter Needs to Know

Available at your local bookstore, or may be ordered by visiting:

Hay House USA: **www.hayhouse.com**®
Hay House Australia: **www.hayhouse.com.au**
Hay House UK: **www.hayhouse.co.uk**
Hay House South Africa: **www.hayhouse.co.za**
Hay House India: **www.hayhouse.co.in**

WOMEN
SEX
POWER&
PLEASURE

GETTING THE LIFE (AND SEX) YOU WANT

EVELYN RESH, MPH, CNM

HAY HOUSE, INC.
Carlsbad, California • New York City
London • Sydney • Johannesburg
Vancouver • Hong Kong • New Delhi

Published and distributed in the United States by: Hay House, Inc.: www .hayhouse.com® • *Published and distributed in Australia by:* Hay House Australia Pty. Ltd.: www.hayhouse.com.au • *Published and distributed in the United Kingdom by:* Hay House UK, Ltd.: www.hayhouse.co.uk • *Published and distributed in the Republic of South Africa by:* Hay House SA (Pty), Ltd.: www.hayhouse.co.za • *Distributed in Canada by:* Raincoast: www.raincoast.com • *Published in India by:* Hay House Publishers India: www.hayhouse.co.in

Cover design: Shelley Noble • *Interior design:* Tricia Breidenthal

The author of this book does not dispense medical advice or pre-scribe the use of any technique as a form of treatment for physical, emo-tional, or medical problems without the advice of a physician, either directly or indirectly. The intent of the author is only to offer information of a general nature to help you in your quest for emotional and spiritual well-being. In the event you use any of the information in this book for yourself, which is your constitutional right, the author and the publisher assume no responsibility for your actions.

Library of Congress Cataloging-in-Publication Data

Resh, Evelyn K., 1959-
  Women, sex, power, and pleasure : getting the life (and sex) you want / Evelyn Resh. -- 1st ed.
      p. cm.
  Includes bibliographical references.
  ISBN 978-1-4019-3631-0 (pbk. : alk. paper) -- ISBN 978-1-4019-3632-7 (ebook) 1. Women--Sexual behavior. 2. Women--Psychology. 3. Sex. 4. Pleasure. I. Title.
  HQ29.R474 2013
  306.7082--dc23
                                                      2012038468

Tradepaper ISBN: 978-1-4019-3631-0
Digital ISBN: 978-1-4019-3632-7

14 15 14 13   4 3 2 1
1st edition, March 2013

Printed in the United States of America

For Robin—
because I love you more

If the world were merely seductive,
that would be easy.
If it were merely challenging,
that would be no problem.
But I arise in the morning
torn between a desire to improve the world
and a desire to enjoy the world.
This makes it hard to plan the day.

E. B. WHITE

CONTENTS

INTRODUCTION

Modern women are amazing. We have high-powered careers, smart kids, terrific partners, lots of exciting friends, beautiful homes, and financial savvy. We seem to know how to manage big money, big responsibilities, and big orgasms with the partners of our choice—and all on our own terms. The exterior is a high-gloss, showy, and impressive pattern with markers of success that women appear to handle effortlessly and with the utmost finesse. But there's so much more to the story. The women who come into my office dispel the myth of the she-has-it-all woman on a daily basis. Beneath this shining exterior, many women are feeling far from successful and are living in *asensual,* sexless relationships, wishing desperately that they actually had the lives we all assume they're leading.

As a sexuality counselor and midwife, this is the side of the story that I see most often. It is in the privacy of my office that the true state of matrimonial unions and the modern American woman's psyche are fully disclosed. I commonly encounter exhausted, furious, overextended wives and mothers who, for all intents and purposes, are tortured by a metastasized lack of pleasure in anything, especially sex. Many face nearly constant battles with their mates because they have disparate appetites for sex, are bored by sex, never liked it in the first place, or can't identify with the idea of its general importance and its relationship to healthy living.

What these women—and possibly you—are missing is not just sex, but pleasure in general. They live lives focused on getting the job done—whatever the job is—and rarely, if ever, take time to enjoy the moment they're in or the pleasures at hand. They also aren't feeling as emotionally healthy and empowered in life as they seem to be to the casual observer, nor do they always speak the truth to some of their closest confidantes.

In order to experience pleasure—in all its forms—our emotional health needs to be sturdy and well integrated into our beings. Genuine self-esteem, spiritual satisfaction, health-seeking behaviors, resilience, creativity, and compassion ignite and sustain our interest in, capability to, and enthusiasm for leading a life filled with pleasure and the sensuality and sexuality associated with it. When seeds of antipleasure are sown either early in life by well-intentioned parents or if our emotional well-being isn't sturdy for whatever reason, our relationships with pleasurable activities—sexual and otherwise—can be anemic. If further cultivated by the demands of career, family, and a drive for accomplishment, then integrating pleasure becomes the pastime and pursuit of only vacationers and underachievers. Pleasure—in and out of bed—has gotten a bad reputation among career-minded, married, and mothering women, and their intimate relationships are showing the wear.

The old but persistent voices of disapproving parents, shabby self-images, complicated sexual histories, limited sexual knowledge, and fatigue can all deter adult women from embracing pleasure with open arms. And if a woman becomes a mother, maternal obligations and responsibilities become her get-out-of-jail-free card, effectively absolving her from paying attention to her overall pleasure quotient in life.

Women in these binds have often unknowingly misappropriated their commitments to themselves and their intimate partners, giving priority instead to their professional worlds and their children. They have lost track of the pleasure they once had, including the pleasure they had with their sexual mates. They become sexually sedate and don't even notice what's missing. Then, sex ends up being just one more thing on their to-do lists. After years of subterranean sexuality, they acclimate to a pleasureless and sexless life, and when anyone brings this to their attention, the tension becomes untenable or all hell breaks loose.

A less than satisfying sex life, or the lack of one altogether, is one of the most painful manifestations of a loss of pleasure, and it's also one of the touchiest subjects to address. When our partners ask for more sex—or any sex, for that matter, perhaps by noting that it's been two weeks, two months, or even two years since you made love, kissed passionately, or slept skin to skin—within milliseconds we turn into she-devils right before our beloveds' eyes, spewing forth the barbed commentary, "Is that all you want from me? *Sex?!* How can you ask for such a thing, after all I do for you, for this family, and in my job?" What I know with certainty from listening to so many women's stories is that when women are pissed off, tired, and estranged from life's pleasures in all forms, we won't put out sexually. It's simply not in our biological makeup to do so, nor does it jibe with our complicated psyches.

When these scenarios show up in my office, I always wait to see just how disturbed the expression on a woman's face becomes when I make note of the fact that what she does for her family, career, and friends falls into a different category from what she does in the name of a healthy sexual relationship or a healthy relationship with herself. Much to her dismay, and sometimes at the risk of enraging her, I become the first and only person to point out that all three relationships are not equal or synonymous. Are they related? Yes, but we're talking apples and oranges and pears.

A woman's self-appointed mandates, tasks, jobs, or obligations have more to do with choice than she often realizes—and for the most part they have almost nothing to do with the maintenance of genuine emotional wellness. They're also frequently a by-product of an anemic relationship with life's pleasures. As a sexuality counselor and a woman who believes that flirting with hedonism is one of the best and most important parts of life, what I look for is just how unhealthy, unpleasant, and therefore unsexy the life of that woman is. There is nothing sexy about being busy every single moment of your day and telling people you like it this way. There's also no way to find any form of pleasure if you have low self-esteem or are experiencing a spiritual crisis, hating your body, feeling like you just can't come back into who you are, or losing all of your creative juices. And let's not even start on the drain your lifestyle has on your compassion and empathy over the long haul. Living this sort of life completely squelches one of the greatest sources of pleasure—and one of the strongest aphrodisiacs of all—being present in the moment and giving your undivided attention to yourself or your mate.

Women of all ages often mistake pleasure for happiness. While experiencing happiness may be related, it's not the same thing as experiencing pleasure. Pleasure-seeking practices contribute to and fortify happiness, but they are also distinctly different from happiness itself. Pleasure is an in-body state but happiness isn't predicated on sensory input and sensate response. They do have an intimate, sometimes dovetailed relationship, but they are not identical or even synonymous. Pleasure by definition includes sensuality. Happiness does not. This is a critical distinction.

Synonyms for pleasure—*comfort, gratification, satisfaction, spice, ease,* and *contentment*—are all words more likely to trigger recollections of feeling states initiated by sensory input before abstract or concrete thinking begins. It may seem counterintuitive that physical pleasure would necessarily precede happiness as opposed to occurring simultaneously. But all thoughts begin with sensory input, and from there we build our scaffold of cognitive knowledge. Then, we formulate thoughts, ideas, and opinions about what we experienced through and within our bodies. Expose someone to a negative sensory input and they're likely to develop negative thoughts about that specific stimulus and things associated with it. The reverse is true with a pleasant sensory experience. Patterns and experiences of exposure result in our own unique biophysical structure of memory with dense layers of recall. We then, consciously and unconsciously, refer to this when we repeat our contact and engagement with pleasing or displeasing stimuli. This continues throughout our lives.

As infants and children we have little if any control over what we come in contact with, but as adults we often have full access to loads of pleasant stimuli. Yet few of us take much advantage of it. We often categorize sensually pleasing experiences as occasional indulgences and rewards for accomplishments rather than practices necessary for maintaining good physical and mental health.

Interestingly, most people don't identify the capacity to experience sensory-mediated pleasures as an inherent feature of personal power. But without our physical bodies and what they allow us to feel, we wouldn't be who we are. And being our real selves is the most powerful thing we can do because it allows us to get the most out of life. The truth of this rarely dawns on us until our physical capacities are diminished or absent due to illness or injury. Then, feelings of impotence and the loss of self-agency can overcome us and make us feel deeply disempowered, if not bereft.

There is currently an entire industry based on helping people feel happy but rarely, if ever, have I seen a discussion on the value of pleasure, sensuality, and sexuality as part of the matrix of factors that contributes to women's happiness and joy. Strange, isn't it? Yet countless times in my practice as a sexuality counselor and midwife—and in my own life—I have seen that when pleasure is nowhere to be found, neither is happiness.

My intention with this book is to use a new lens to examine why modern women are so alienated from pleasure in general. I'll look at why women say no to sex so often when they're in loving relationships with men and women they tell me they're attracted to and want to have sex with more often. I hope to reacquaint women with what it means to have real emotional well-being up and running in their daily lives and how doing so leads to more powerful and pleasurable living—and to increased interest in and access to sex.

Each chapter you'll read is written from four perspectives: those of an experienced midwife, a sexuality counselor, a happily married middle-aged woman, and a mother. Based on my experiences as a sexuality counselor and as a flawed, 50-something gal, my views on what keeps a woman's drive for pleasure and sex intact over time comes from the dilemmas my patients describe and the mishaps in my own life. I don't have all the answers, a magic pill, or a precise prescription to cure you of the blahs. I am not a psychotherapist, marriage counselor, doctor, or sexpert, but I do know what it's like to deal with the trials and tribulations of keeping pleasure and sex alive. I have also had the extraordinary privilege of talking with hundreds of women and men about what sex means to them and what they feel are obstacles to finding the sexual pleasure they want.

At the end of chapters 2 through 7 you will find questions to ask yourself that may help you understand more about your own difficulties with giving sex and pleasure a palpable pulse and audible respirations in your own life and relationships. And trust me, these really are questions I have asked myself before—sometimes on a daily basis.

We're all works in progress, forever seeking new truths and greater self-insight to make life sweeter. But gaining insight doesn't always have to be painful, protracted, and somber. In fact, as you cozy up to read, prepare yourself for advice given with levity and daring from the real-life and honest, well-intentioned voice of a seeker of the magic formula. I also love sex and hope to be able to say so— in earnest—forever. Make no mistake about it: I am right there with you.

CHAPTER 1

THE MARKERS OF EMOTIONAL WELL-BEING

"Well-being is just like 'weather' or 'freedom' in its structure: no single measure defines it exhaustively, but several things contribute to it . . . "

—MARTIN SELIGMAN

Today is a perfect New England spring day. This is a real gift after more than a week of cloudy skies and intermittent intense rainfall that has flooded basements and dampened spirits. My second-floor study has a small window that faces our driveway, making it easy for me to hear the cars and trucks that occasionally go up and down our country road. I heard the truck coming before anyone else in the house did. It was the landscaper with our delivery. Beautiful, rich loam, here in time to plant our garden before Memorial Day—what a pleasure! I know a truck full of dirt wouldn't be high on everyone's wish list. But when your heart is in your garden, a big pile of new loam is a dream come true. It smells right, feels good on your hands, looks just right, and will lay the foundation for a garden filled with the flowers and vegetables we love most. The pleasure in that new loam will last for a long time and will lead me to other pleasures, if I allow it to.

Pleasure begets pleasure. The soothing or enlivening effects of pleasurable stimuli have a way of reminding us of our capacity to take something simple—like new loam—and transform it into a reparative unguent or restorative tonic. Pleasures, if taken throughout the day, support our emotional immunity and fortify our ability to combat the cavalcades of stressors and disappointments that are common in life. Frequent pleasurable interludes and pick-me-ups improve our overall resilience by interrupting the physical manifestations of stress (e.g., stiff muscles, headaches, indigestion) and replacing them with something that feels good and is better for us. The subsequent cognitive and in-the-flesh memories of these pleasurable sensations build upon themselves—pleasure begets pleasure—making the route to pleasure easier to find and more appealing. The more we have, the more we want. My capacity to access and experience pleasurable things also makes me feel empowered to enjoy life simply because of who I am—in body and mind—independent of anyone else's actions or opinions. I say this to myself every day. It is my mantra, my prayer, my incantation for sweet living, decadent relaxation, meaningful productivity, and satisfying sex. The connection is rooted in my moving from one pleasure to another with deliberation, every day, and placing a high value on doing so consistently. Accomplishing this depends on my having good emotional health; this is what piques my interest in pleasurable living in the first place, allows me access to it, and keeps me coming back for more. Emotional well-being equals powerful living, which equals increased interest and access to pleasure of all kinds. This, in turn, leads to improved mental health, and the cycle repeats. Without emotional well-being, none of us can locate, engage in, or benefit from any of the pleasures that life has to offer—and sex is not an exception.

Women talk to me about how busy they are *all the time*. Nearly everyone I know is trying to gain balance between work and rest, productivity and downtime, and caring for others and practicing sustainable self-care. I am all for these efforts to balance our obligations with leisure activities. Yet, when we talk about the benefits of gaining equilibrium in life we rarely, if ever, hear about how doing so will impact our ability to access pleasure or our sexuality. Despite the vast number of titles available on how to increase your happiness quotient in life—all of which claim to have the real definition of happiness for everyone—the bestsellers in this genre almost never mention satisfying sex as a part of a pleasurable and rewarding life. What is going on here?

Women's roles in society over the last half century have changed dramatically. More women than ever are graduating from college, earning more money than men, and choosing to postpone having children on behalf of their professional development. With better educations, higher incomes, and greater autonomy, we should have an unending list of pleasurable things and activities that reads like a soup-to-nuts assortment of delights. But based on my experience as a sexuality counselor and midwife, women's lives are often more complicated and taxing than they are pleasant. Many of the women I care for spend a dispro-portionate amount of time focused on their productivity at work and at home. They don't even consider doing some-thing pleasant. And while we may have more money than ever to spend on a mani-pedi and fancy yoga clothes, we often do so while arguing on our cell phones with kids and co-workers who aren't doing things the "right" way. So much for relaxing, pleasurable pampering. Despite such improved circumstances, loads of women complain about not having the time and energy to do what pleases them most. They also confess details of their mediocre or non-existent sex lives with taciturn expressions they hope will disguise both their sulfuric rage and their deep, sometimes unrelenting heartache.

Concern over women's interest in sex—or lack of it—has been a hot topic in the hallowed halls of medicine and the media over the past 15 years. According to medical experts, 26 to 43 percent of American women complain of having a decreased or absent sex drive.[1] This is true for women of all ages, although the percentage may be even higher in postmenopausal women. True to form, the American public has looked to the medical establishment for answers. All medicine has managed to come up with thus far is a billable diagnosis: hypoactive sexual desire disorder (HSDD). This is described by the *Diagnostic and Statistical Manual of Mental Disorders* as a lack of interest in sex, which is what women and their partners already knew they were struggling with. No discovery or medi-cal breakthrough here. And although in my own practice I sometimes prescribe certain hormones for patients whose libidos have completely hit the skids or for those who used to be orgasmic but now rarely or never are, only a very small percentage of the women I care for fit the criteria for pharmaceutical intervention as a fix.

Books in the how-to-have-better-sex genre mimic international cookbooks in their diversity and flavor. The overly enthusiastic, misinformed (and sometimes cruel) "you can do it!" coaching approach, the "light the candles and wear sexy lingerie" prescription, and the "your brain is your biggest sex organ" theory do little to help women flip their switches to wanting sex more often and prioritizing it over the long run. They also fail to recommend ways to manage the frequently absurd and humorous interventions by Murphy's Law that seem to govern life and undo our best-laid plans for fabulous, romantic, sizzling sex with our partners.

I think about this all the time. This is not because I am a sex fiend, whore, promulgator of pornography, pervert, or weirdo. I think about it because it's a complex problem that I try to solve for myself and on behalf of the women (and men) I care for in my sex counseling practice. This is meaningful stuff that, if left untended, can break our hearts, leave us feeling stranded and unloved, and perhaps destroy long-term relationships.

When I feel at a loss for an explanation as to why sexual energy is nowhere to be found in my own life, I go back to my belief that pleasure begets pleasure and that in order to increase my pleasure quotient I need to feel powerful. I begin there and work the equation forward: emotional wellness equals powerful living equals increased interest and access to all pleasures, including sex. Then I ask myself just how sturdy and powerful I'm feeling. If the answer is "not very," then I need to figure out why. When I apply this to the women I see for sexuality counseling, I start by asking the same questions: How is your emotional health? How empowered do you feel to get what you really want?

How much pleasure are you able to surround yourself with and what might be interfering with that? If their emotional health is weak or an aspect of it has always been anemic, then this is probably why their interest in sex is absent. In this state it's nearly impossible to grab and keep hold of pleasure, breaking the stride of the pleasure-begets-pleasure formula.

Women who struggle with having consistent interest in sex or finding sex pleasurable when they do have it can gain insight into why this is so by seriously considering how powerful they feel as people and how willing they are to prioritize their emotional health. The answers to these two questions are inextricably linked to six markers of emotional well-being that I feel are critical for good mental health: self-confidence and self-esteem, health-seeking behaviors, spiritual satisfaction, creativity, resilience, and compassion. The strength of these markers will determine your feelings of empowerment and capacity to prioritize and safeguard pleasure. When these are sturdy and unyielding, your appetite for *all* pleasure will be robust and your ability to prioritize it will be securely woven into the fabric of your psyche. In contrast, when these markers have been ignored or tipped over for long periods of time, or were never upright in the first place, none of life's pleasures—including sex—may ever exist in their real-life forms.

Women face all sorts of demands in the course of a single day. Responsibilities pile up throughout the weeks, months, and years and become weighty yokes around our necks. Sometimes, the effort it takes to pull them off can feel like more work than continuing to lug them around. Every time we try to shorten our to-do lists, something else seems to take the place of the things we were able to unload. Before we know it, we're right back where we started and life continues as one big, blurry, snarled mess of obligations and tasks. And, lest we believe we can sneak away and get a real break from it all, our technological devices, designed to help us save time, end up seducing us right back to our to-do lists. Based on my professional and personal experience, living life the way so many of us do is a real harbinger of death to our libidos and a surefire way to distract and estrange us from maintaining our emotional wellness.

My sex counseling and midwifery practices are replete with women who tell me that if they never have sex again they wouldn't care or even notice. These are women who also say they love their mates, want to stay with them forever, and cannot imagine life without them. Yet somehow, the idea of making love with them often—or at all—leaves them flat and filled with a sense of dread. Hard to fathom that both feelings can coexist, and yet women tell me all the time that they do.

When I scratch the surface of their complaints, the picture that starts to emerge is of a life filled with everything but pleasure. Without fail, one if not all of the six markers of emotional well-being are off-kilter. Maybe they lack confidence, hate their bodies, or do nothing to support a healthy lifestyle. Perhaps they've lost their faith and optimism because of the recent death of someone they loved or health problems of their own. Or, maybe they've lost their creative edge and can't find meaning in their work anymore, which threatens their identity. And, there's always the possibility that they're unable to recover from a mistake—theirs or someone else's—which can mean they've lost compassion for themselves or someone else. Usually, at least one if not all of these factors are present, and if they are, sexuality will be absent no matter how much they love and are attracted to their partners.

Let's look more closely at the six markers of emotional well-being. If we understand these well, we'll see just how important they are to our sense of enjoyment in life, love, and sex.

MARKER 1: SELF-ESTEEM AND SELF-CONFIDENCE

The self-help genre is based on the "love thyself" motto. With millions of titles now in print, anyone would be hard-pressed to find one that doesn't stress the importance of loving oneself as a precedent for loving all others. Personally, I am not convinced that looking in the mirror daily and saying I love you to my reflection (and meaning it all the time) is necessary to feel deep and genuine love for my family and friends. However, I do know unequivocally that our opinions of ourselves directly influence our ability and willingness to live self-empowered and pleasurable lives every day—and to take our personal enjoyment seriously. This includes the pleasure we feel from the compliments and loving gestures made by those we do love and who love us back.

Concluding that you're an idiot, ass, jerk, or moron is bound to happen hundreds of times throughout life. Whether or not you're actually right about this is really beside the point. Feeling this way in any given moment is enough to make it so—at least temporarily. Welcome to the business of living. Invariably something or someone will come along and point out to you that you've failed at something you tried to master; that someone whose features are the opposite of yours is beautiful; or that despite putting your best foot forward, you're simply not cutting the mustard. Questioning your self-worth, confidence, or your true strengths because of a specific circumstance or situation you happened to land in is one thing. All of us do this. And in moderation it represents the critically important capacity for self-reflection that can hone your self-insight. The resultant clarity of preference and purpose actually boosts your self-esteem and can leave you feeling what I call *sexy smart*. In other words, you're a woman who knows what she wants and goes for it. There is nothing sexier than self-confidence, which doesn't depend on how much you weigh, how many gray hairs you have, or how much money you make. This was nicely summed up by one of my clients, who explained how her self-confidence and self-respect carried her through a difficult time and kept her feeling sexy and appealing:

> Despite how rough things had gotten at work, I kept reminding myself of how smart people had told me I was and that I would land on my feet. Really, I had the wind at my back, even though it didn't seem that way on first pass. Despite being fucked over and struggling with a difficult boss and an unexpected situation, I held my head high and relied on my genuine knowing of what I was capable. Hanging on to my essential self-confidence helped me stay balanced and confident, despite the way I was being treated. I didn't let myself feel downtrodden, and I never ended up feeling that people looked at me that way, either. —*Elaine, 52*

In contrast, women who feel like idiots and stay stuck in this feeling aren't insightful, nor do they ever feel or think sexy smart; they loathe themselves, and this has seriously negative and predictably grave consequences. Furthermore, there is nothing sexy about it. Compare the following statement to the one above and you'll see what I mean:

> Even though I have lost weight, improved my health and fitness, can look in the mirror and feel good about my appearance, *and* was the one who decided to leave my marriage, I have no real confidence that I will ever meet anyone else or that anyone will ever find me attractive or smart enough to want to date me. I have this self-hatred that just won't quit, no matter what I do in the name of self-improvement. I can laugh about it a lot of the time, but truly, inside it's an ongoing, constant ache. —*Julia, 41*

Women who dislike themselves no matter what they accomplish and always find fault with who they are bear a terrible burden. They can't find anything about themselves they truly like, respect, or admire. Consequentially, they don't feel powerful enough to access what they honestly want out of life and their relationships. Women who feel this way also find it very difficult to think of themselves as sexual beings and to imagine themselves as sexually appealing. No matter how often their partners tell them they're attractive or express desire for them, self-loathing women will spurn their advances and retreat into never-ending lists of distracting tasks and chores in the hopes that accomplishing them will boost their egos. This is an onerous, self-defeating process that robs the afflicted of more and more pleasure as time goes on. Women who live in self-loathing have only brief interludes of pleasure and these are unsustainable and difficult to replicate on a frequent basis. These are my patients who can't make lists of things they find pleasurable when I ask them to. The cumulative effect of their lack of self-confidence is pernicious and erodes their receptivity and ability to detect pleasure in even the most obviously pleasurable things. It becomes a self-feeding and self-fulfilling system with a strong and deadly undertow.

And women don't need to hate everything about themselves for self-loathing to have this cloying, erosive effect. Even if there is just one particular thing a woman hates about herself, she can end up spending time in her own version of perdition with nonstop references to that one thing. In these situations, all roads lead back to the feature or characteristic she loathes, no matter how closely related it is or isn't to her perceived success or failure. The expanse and depth of loathing are the issue, not the specific feeling of loathing itself.

MARKER 2: HEALTH-SEEKING BEHAVIORS

The definition of *healthy living* is the ongoing subject of magazine articles, reality television shows, and self-help books that attract people's attention like flies to flypaper. Despite the particulars of the debate, it's a given that a diet of Milk Duds, soda, and corn chips in combination with a sedentary lifestyle, smoking, and heavy drinking will likely land you in the Chubby Department, cardiac unit, and on insulin much faster than if you're a nonsmoking, vegetarian hiking enthusiast. As a health-care provider who is well informed about the value of making healthy choices and a middle-aged realist who is easily undermined by her sweet tooth and love of leisure, what I strive for in my own life and look for in the lives of my patients is approximately an 80–20 split. I urge women to participate in health-seeking behaviors approximately 80 percent of the time; the rest is up for grabs. And, perhaps even more important, I encourage them to understand that this is a reasonable and realistic approach to living a good life. When women either aim for 100 percent compliance with one presumed gold standard for health or ignore them all completely, the results are equally damaging to their psyches—and their sex lives.

Sad but true, we live in a polluted world and one that is filled with daily opportunities to distract ourselves from eating well, exercising, and sleeping enough. I advise my patients (and I make an effort myself) to buy organic foods, exercise three to five times weekly for an hour or so, never smoke, have regular health screenings, and not compromise their seven to eight hours of sleep each night. I also sometimes happily eat cookies for dinner, prune my sleep time in favor of watching a good movie, and have sex in the middle of the afternoon instead of exercising. The way I see it, humans have built-in limitations, including an expiration date. None of us will leave here alive, but we are all masters of how we spend our time while we're here. I love so many of life's pleasures and I do my best to maintain habits that I hope will maximize my chances for enjoying them for as long as possible. But, I also hedge my bets 20 percent of the time and let the sky be the limit on pleasure for pleasure's sake.

Talking with a woman who is convinced her world will stop in its orbit if she eats a pint of ice cream once in a while—just because she loves it—is just as worrisome to me as a woman who tells me without pause that she drinks a half bottle of red wine nightly because it's good for her heart. When women function on either end of the behavioral continuum, it reveals an unrealistic attitude toward health, and both extremes impair and distort their experience of pleasure—the first because of rigidity, the second because of foolhardy denial.

I once worked with a woman who came to me for preconceptual counseling. She and her husband were planning to start a family in the near future and she wanted to discuss the optimal diet and exercise plan for conception and pregnancy. I began our conversation by asking her what and how she ate. She was quite lean, and I had the suspicion that she had a history of an eating disorder. She admitted that my suspicions were correct, but added that this had been "resolved" and was no longer a problem. I was doubtful and with good reason. As it turned out, her intake of carbohydrates was dangerously low. The average person needs a minimum of 100 grams of carbohydrates per day for normal brain function, and from her report, she wasn't anywhere near this daily requirement. She also wasn't getting enough fats or protein. Her overall calorie intake, even with the additional 300 calories needed to sustain a pregnancy, would still be less than optimal. When I explained this to her, she became very anxious and told me that what I was proposing as an alternative way of eating sounded excessive and not doable for her. Despite this being in the best interests of fetal growth and her own health, it was clear that such a deviation from what she perceived to be healthy eating was beyond her emotional tolerance. This is a stunning example of how rigidity can eclipse common sense and logic, even when the stakes are so high.

In contrast, there are women who have no concept of restraint and put their health at risk because of blind excess. I have spoken to many women about their drinking habits and have found them to be astonishingly misinformed about—and unwilling to accept—what is considered moderate drinking.

According to the National Institute on Alcohol Abuse and Alcoholism, moderate alcohol consumption for women is 12 ounces of beer, 1.5 ounces of hard liquor, or a 5-ounce glass of wine per day.[2] In case you're wondering how much wine that actually is, it's one-half cup plus a splash. Frankly, I don't know anyone who drinks that amount of wine when they pour it themselves or order it in a restaurant. The "wine as medicine" idea is popular with women, and vintners have even incorporated this concept into their labeling. The fact that brands such as Mommy's Time Out and MommyJuice exist at all tells us something about women's use of wine for relaxation and restoration of the mind and body. This has come through loud and clear when I have counselled one of the many women who *must have* their merlot or chardonnay at the end of a long and demanding day. As one woman, who was drinking about three 8- to 10-ounce glasses of wine each night, put it to me: "If you're about to tell me that I drink too much, don't go there. I don't agree. I have heart disease in my family and high blood pressure and I am sure this is helping to prevent both. And anyway, this is not a negotiable issue. I am not giving up one of my few enjoyments in life, even if I do drink a bit more than I should sometimes." I certainly wouldn't want her to be driving me home after she had had her fill.

Then there are the many women I counsel who have developed exercise routines that are more likely to break their bodies down than build them up and keep them strong. These women aren't able to reconcile skipping a day at the gym; they will forfeit needed sleep and run instead or skip the pleasure of a social outing to exercise because they think they'll get fat.

Counseling women with dietary, exercise, or drinking habits driven by anxiety, body hate, or difficulty in coping with stress is like watching Theatre of the Absurd—normal human behaviors and needs become nefarious enemies one must attack or avoid. And, things can get more complex; if you can't enjoy moving safely and in moderation or eating and drinking with gusto and sensibility, you're highly unlikely to be interested in sex or any other body-based pleasure. If you have a massage, you'll be wondering how the therapist can stand to touch you because your body is just so disgusting. Shopping for new clothes will be a ring of *Dante's Inferno* and every meal will have the potential to become a caloric crisis. And, your lover(s) will take the worst beating of all when you sequester your body completely from his or her longing gaze and well-intentioned hands. There is no self-empowerment or pleasure-begetting-pleasure model at work here—just a dangerous downward spiral.

MARKER 3: SPIRITUAL SATISFACTION

I define healthy and intact spirituality for myself and my clients as a combination of optimism and faith. It's that simple. While these two concepts are highly subjective and sometimes easily misunderstood, they're unmistakable to most of us when they're absent. I picture spirituality in my mind's eye as a double helix—one strand faith, the other optimism, each curving around the other to form one solid ribbon. I think of it as the DNA of the soul. People who have lost their optimism and faith will tell you they feel emotionally bankrupt. They're adrift, feel that they have nothing to hold on to, and do not feel self-empowered. This is a terrible state, and it's reflective of what happens when our feelings of positivity and hope have evaporated.

When I was growing up in the 1960s, '70s, and '80s, talk of your spirituality never made it into regular, everyday conversations. Back in those days, being *spiritual* meant being a religious insurgent or nut. And frankly, there was some truth to this considering the cast of notorious religious leaders of the times: the Reverend Jim Jones, Jim and Tammy Faye Bakker, Sun Myung Moon, Charles Manson, and let's not forget the Hare Krishna. All these folks made spirituality their platform with some bizarre and deadly outcomes. Needless to say, this left the majority of us non-converts suspicious of and worried about spirituality—at the very least.

Fast-forward 30 years. We now have an entire industry based on spiritual enlightenment and health. This new and profitable corner of American commerce creates products designed to enhance, fortify, protect, and advance your spirituality and your spiritual identity. Spiritual health and beliefs are often the topic of people's conversations these days, especially if they're candidates for public office.

The scientific community has even gotten in on the game with studies exploring the impact of spiritual states on literal brain function and overall health. Sophisticated scans like MRIs and PETs now allow the viewing and measuring of actual brain activity. These scanners have been able to prove that subjects deep in meditation and prayer have altered brain functioning that positively influences certain health markers such as blood pressure, pulse rate, respiration rate, and mood. Surely the knowledge of these scans' results must impact the feelings of optimism and faith of those devoted to a daily meditation practice or the devout who pray for the salvation of their souls and God's mercy for the world's sinners.

My concern in this area of well-being is not what type of spirituality a person has, but rather if they have one at all, leaving it wide open for the atheists, agnostics, and everyone in between. Folks don't need to believe in a divine power, being, or afterlife. All I am looking for is a

declaration of optimism and faith that comes from somewhere or something.

Regardless of your personal opinion about the definition of spirituality, when someone loses their feelings of
faith and optimism about life, chances are high that their
pleasure quotient has also hit rock bottom. These are folks
who have a noteworthy if not discouraging disempowered
attitude about life's outcomes: "I have no control over what
happens anyway. What's going to happen will happen."
Call me a simpleton, but I feel like I have plenty of power
and control to affect outcomes in my life, and my faith and
optimism play a major role in this. I am not a blind optimist,
but I am reticent to absolve myself of any influence what-
soever over how my life progresses. Those who embrace an
abject attitude of surrender are actively cultivating a mindset antithetical to the value of pleasure to body, mind, and
empowered living. This also reflects a belief that pleasurable experiences are not palliative, therapeutic, valuable, or
influential in any way. They don't care about pleasure and
they frequently couldn't care less about having sex. Really,
what would be the point? Consider the story below from
a woman who came to me about the loss of her sexual energy. To me, this was a clear case of a spiritual crisis inciting
a loss of all things pleasurable:

> My best friend from childhood died about nine
> months ago. She had been diagnosed with pancreatic
> cancer and didn't live long after the diagnosis. She was
> only 39! She had two young children and a lovely hus-
> band. She was the last person I ever would have imag-
> ined would get something like that—always exercised,
> ate organic food, was really conscientious about her
> health. It's left me feeling like no matter what you do, it
> doesn't matter. If this can happen to her, it can happen

to anyone. Since her death I have become a real fatalist about everything, and I feel as though all my best intentions in life don't matter. If she can die at 39, then what's going to stop anything like that from happening to me? I have no faith in anything anymore, and I certainly don't feel optimistic about anything in life. —*Celia, 38*

Self-empowerment, pleasure, and spiritual satisfaction are intricately linked, and sex comes next. In order to feel powerful, enjoy pleasurable things, and be receptive to sexual intimacy, you simply have to have the faith and optimism necessary to see a good thing when it's standing right in front of you. This is the biggest problem you'll face if your spiritual satisfaction goes asunder. It sets off a chain reaction of negative thinking that eclipses its more pleasurable and neurologically healthy, mood-lifting opposite.

MARKER 4: CREATIVITY

My ability to cultivate new ideas, interpret what my clients are saying with enthusiasm and quick, accurate analysis, and write with enjoyment are all diagnostically significant; they mean my creative juices are flowing and I'm functioning optimally. I am humming along, feeling powerful, and continually living a pleasurable life as a result. This is so true for me that when the well runs dry and I haven't had an original idea for weeks or months, I know that I need to radically change something in my life— figuratively and literally.

Talking about being creative with clients can initially be confusing. They wonder if I am asking what sort of art or craft they do. You don't need to be a fine-arts person or do crafts to be creative. Creativity is whatever you do that identifies you to others, infuses your life with meaning, and lets you sign your name to things in bold script. This can include your professional work, but gardening, baking and cooking, sewing, planning parties, singing, and playing an instrument all count, too. These are all valid examples of how creativity manifests in people's lives. When you engage in these pursuits, you'll feel sturdy in your identity and others will notice. In fact, they'll easily recognize you. And when they don't, they'll say things like "You just don't seem like yourself" and it's because you really aren't. This is how one of my clients explained it to me:

> I felt as though I was slowly dying in the job I just left. My position became less and less creative and much more administrative. That's not what I want from my work. I need to be able to use my imagination and my people skills in combination with each other to feel satisfied with what I'm doing. I was withering, and I could feel it affecting every aspect of my life; my memory and concentration were poor, I started to feel depressed, I stopped cooking meals, and my relationship with my partner was negatively affected. The longer I stayed there, the less I felt like myself. —*Gwen, 44*

New research on creativity and the creative mind is all good news. The more engaged your mind is in all sorts of things, the more likely you are to have one that works properly and for longer. If you knit, keep it up. Do crossword puzzles, play sudoku, read biographies, watch birds, and go to continuing education classes. If you do, your brain will capitalize on its ability to expand at the microscopic level even while it's shrinking in overall size with normal aging.

My clients who are artists—painters, writers, actresses, dancers—rely on their creativity as real life-force energy. My Middle Eastern dance teacher, Carmen Davis, has a framed poster in her studio that says: "You ask: why do I dance; why do I breathe?" Watching Carmen dance is an extraordinary experience. She is captivating, so talented, and radiantly authentic. Carmen is deeply familiar with the importance of creativity in her life. She has breathed through dance for over 45 years because it continually re-affirms her identity and gives her life a sense of meaning.

We all have talents that make us who we are and give us purpose in life. Without them, our identities dwindle and we lose our individuality. This couldn't help but rattle your emotional well-being, feelings of self-empowerment, and ability to access pleasure.

MARKER 5: RESILIENCE

The qualities of resilience and self-confidence are intimately related, but they are distinct enough that I feel it's important to talk about both. The difference lies in how you react when something doesn't go your way. Self-confident people can move forward with vigor and presence, but if they aren't also resilient they could be brought down by failure. Resilience is the ability to reassure yourself that you'll manage somehow, even when life's events diverge and move in unexpected or unintended directions.

Resilient, self-assured women are easily able to acknowledge what they don't know or aren't good at, take it in stride (given that we can't be good at everything), and then ask someone for help without experiencing this as a threat to their ego, self-esteem, or sense of identity.

This is impossible for women who are fundamentally insecure and have a distorted sense of competence. When the über-competent, insecure woman bumps up against something difficult or impossible for her to master, it can feel unbearable. This can be said about many of today's modern, well-educated, professional gals who have impressive capabilities in so many areas. But when they hit the wall because of something that's beyond them or are outwitted by something, they find it very difficult to ride the wave.

My professional life has been split between extremes of the population. Part of the time I care for girls and women who are intellectually, culturally, and economically disadvantaged. Many are in the class of the working poor in this country, and they aren't well educated, barely make it from paycheck to paycheck, and have little hope of ever improving their lot in life. Simultaneously, I care for upper-class and very wealthy women who are well-educated professionals with luxurious lives, plenty of money, and resources of all kinds. The two groups are so different and yet, women in the latter group suffer from an inner turmoil I almost never see in the other population. The rich and resourceful have difficulty reassuring themselves when they can't completely control or manage something. They're often so accustomed to successfully orchestrating their lives and arranging things *exactly* the way they want them that when they face something out of their control or beyond their skill set, they can find it impossible to come to terms with. Interestingly, even with all the things they've learned and mastered, they haven't really had the need or opportunity to hone their resilience, and when facing personal limitations they feel like they're at risk for losing face. These women have a very low tolerance for disappointment. They can reach an emotional breaking point when they can't lose the last ten pounds of pregnancy weight after delivery, discover their child is only moderately above average intelligence, have gray hair coming in, or are given a medical diagnosis like infertility. These kinds of things unravel them and lead them to question their self-worth, literally. Being unable to conquer, vanquish, or control something is a personal failing, a black mark on their reputations and overall value. Not being good at something or not being able to control a situation is not simply "one of those things" in life. Consider these comments from two of my patients:

> I have always been health conscious. I only eat organic food, I watch my weight, and my periods are regular. I cannot believe that I can't get pregnant! Maybe I'm just not going to the right specialists. I know lots of women who have gotten pregnant at 41—I think we just need to find a better doctor. I can't accept that I can't get pregnant and have a child of my own. I waited so long to make sure that I would have everything I needed to do this "right," and now they're telling me I can't conceive for unexplained reasons; everything can be explained! My husband has talked to me about either adopting or not having children at all and has said that it's me he wants more than anything, but I can't accept this. I'm sure he's going to leave me for someone else, despite what he says. —Sharon, 41

> I cannot stand this change in my body since menopause. No matter what I do, I cannot lose this belly fat, and I never had any fat on my belly before. I have talked to my gynecologist, my personal trainer, and my yoga teacher about this and they've all said that there is a redistribution of fat with aging and menopause and that even nonoverweight women will have this, but I refuse

to accept that there isn't something that can be done about it. If I can't get rid of it with exercise and dieting, I'll have surgery. I am not living with this. It's ugly and I hate it and it makes me hate everything about my body. I feel like people are staring at that no matter what I'm wearing. I don't care if I'm healthy and in good shape. I don't care what the experts say or what the risks of elective surgery are. I will have it anyway—anything to get rid of this fat. —Joyce, 54

Dwindling fertility and postmenopausal belly fat are hardly the determinants of poor, weak, or suspicious character. But, when natural forces can capsize your ego and sense of worth and you can't come back at them with any humility, grace, or humor, then it's highly unlikely that you feel particularly resilient, and certainly not powerful. And as far as easily accessing life's pleasures and having sex, just forget about it!

MARKER 6: COMPASSION AND EMPATHY

I have the true good fortune of living in a small, rural farming community in the hills of western Massachusetts. This hill country is beautiful, serene, and home to an eclectic group of residents. All of us who live here rely on one another and help out when the need arises. This is unquestionably exemplified by the work of our volunteer fire and ambulance crews.

I had a bizarre accident one morning while hiking in our local woods. I slipped on wet leaves and fell, and a branch impaled my left arm. Later that night, I added insult to injury by having a seizure, an adverse effect from the pain medication I had taken. My terrified partner called 911 and our neighbor, both of whom arrived within moments, to cart me out of the house and back to the hospital. I am almost certain that our neighbor and ambulance team members would have preferred to continue watching television at 9 P.M. rather than manage my medical emergency. But genuine compassion for others isn't shadowed by personal preference. That's one of its distinguishing features. When compassion is at work your personal comfort and convenience aren't in the foreground of your thinking. Your objective is to give and be kind to others. This is a deeply self-empowering tool, and it leads to an infusion of pleasure that's long lasting and meaningful and strengthens your emotional connections to others.

If you have ever sat with someone who lacks compassion and empathy—I refer to it as "the longest lunch of your life!"—you have probably found them to be positively insufferable. People who lack compassion manage to turn every spotlight back onto themselves. They also will forever have a reason for their lack of availability to do something for someone else and aren't really able to carry out a single act of goodwill on their own. And, if they are generous, it's likely done for personal benefit in the long run, not because it's simply the *right* thing to do. They're the ones who won't drop off a bag of clothes for the poor unless they can get a receipt for their taxes—then, they'll inflate the amount of their donation. When it comes to sexuality, they are deeply disappointing lovers—everything ends up being all about them, even when they say they're trying to please you.

Consider the following statements from three of my clients, each of whose partner's lack of compassion has had a dramatic impact on their sexual relationship.

24

We have been dealing with the fallout from my husband's felony charges for more than five years now, and it has cost us millions of dollars in legal fees. I am so angry, humiliated, and embarrassed by what he's done and the stress on me has been immeasurable. He still wants to have sex often and I just can't fathom it! When I tried to explain to him how being near him in that way just feels impossible and that it's related to all that his actions have put us through, he responded by asking me, "Well how do you think I feel?" I was shocked! How could he have the balls to say that? Who cares how *he* feels, what about how I feel? —*Rachel, 40*

The only way I am able to get my husband to watch our children and give me time to myself is if I agree to have sex with him as payment for his time. We've gone to marriage counselors, and he starts out liking them until they tell him that this trade agreement just isn't a reasonable or kind way to behave. Then, he turns on them and he'll tell me they don't know what they're talking about and that he won't go back to them. I love him and he is the father of my children, but I can't help but feel like I am a sort of sex slave. He's kind in some ways: he'll buy me the things I want, we live in a beautiful house, and he's a good father. But I am just not interested in having sex with him because of this. It makes me feel like a whore and I don't really feel loved. —*Meredith, 42*

Everyone loves my husband and always tells me how lucky I am to be married to him. People always talk about how handsome, funny, and generous he is. But they don't live with him and have no idea what goes on behind closed doors. He's selfish and never thinks about what I might be experiencing and how it affects me.

> When I am sick he dismisses it and doesn't help me with anything in the house or with our kids. But, when he's sick, he demands that I drop everything and take care of him. I am so exhausted! Even when we make love it's all about him. Like for example, he's always asking me if I had an orgasm and when I explain that I don't need to have one to enjoy myself, he tells me there's something wrong with me. He's just not kind to me, and I don't feel like he acts in a loving way toward me. The idea of having sex with him is a turnoff. —*Joan, 38*

A lack of compassion is not gender specific. Read this statement from a client of mine who was struggling with his wife's dispassionate behavior:

> My wife and I were high school sweethearts. We have been together for over 20 years. I am crazy about her, but I have felt less and less important to her since our kids were born. The ranking in her mind is kids, their needs, the house, and me last. No matter what amount of time I ask for with her, she always tells me I am asking for too much and that the kids come first—always. The kids come first. It's not that I don't understand how important children are or how much they rely on their mother. But since our kids were born, I feel . . . deceased. I just don't feel like I matter at all to her. —*James, 38*

While you might not be involved with a felon or a sex-for-trade partner or feel "deceased" because of your partner's neglect, if any of the descriptions in these paragraphs sound like someone you're coupled with, I would think seriously about your choice. Or, if your partner tells you you're like this on a regular basis, I suggest you reflect on that with the help of a skilled professional. Lacking compassion and empathy often stems from deeply rooted feelings of insecurity that have contorted into a terrible, ugly form and make the sufferer very hard to love—a fait accompli if there ever was one. There's no way to live a truly self-empowered and pleasurable life under these circumstances, and it's definitely not an aphrodisiac for your partner.

PUTTING IT ALL TOGETHER

So, now that you've taken a tour through the markers of emotional well-being and have a taste of how they can affect and afflict your ability to access pleasure, what can you do to keep them upright? How do we reright them when life's inevitable hits and slams knock us off our feet? Or, what happens if one of these markers has been wobbly for as long as you can remember?

In the next several chapters, I'll look at things we all contend with and how they can disrupt and sometimes dismantle our emotional wellness and powerful lives and why the impact is so forceful and destructive. Then, I'll give you strategies and suggestions for avoiding the hits in the first place and pulling yourself back together when you simply can't help but be the bull's-eye for the poison dart. Trouble will find you—it's just part of being human and living a full life. But trouble doesn't have to destroy your self-empowerment, your relationship with pleasure, or your sexuality. In fact, pleasure in any form is often the antidote to life's hardest hits. And how about learning how to incorporate some preventive measures into your lifestyle so trouble doesn't end up being maximally destructive? Have you ever thought about preventing the loss of your libido as a worthwhile health measure? I am guessing you haven't.

Keep reading and remember that pleasure begets plea-sure—sexual pleasure included—and that when it comes to keeping your pleasure quotient high and your sexuality accessible, you are the master of your own destiny.

CHAPTER 2

I'M JUST
TOO BUSY

It's not so much how busy you are, but why you are busy. The bee is praised. The mosquito is swatted.

—MARY O'CONNOR

Women often tell me that pleasure and sex just feel like one *more* thing to do on their already daunting and lengthy to-do lists. Most women believe that sex should be something that catches them off guard, sweeps them off their feet, and is infused with combusting passion and mutual orgasms worth bragging about. The idea of planning for sex takes the wind out of their sails and feels like a total buzz kill. Apparently, sex should *just happen*—like sneezing. No planning required. I imagine these women see it something like this: there you are just minding your own business, and then sex comes along and decides for you that you'll be overcome by its propulsive force and have no choice but to give in. This is a very strange idea and an ineffective way of trying to have the sex life you want. On the other hand, women also say, "When we do have sex, I always wonder, *Why don't we do this more often?* I feel so great afterward!" At some point in their critical thinking, the interconnectedness of satisfying sex and active participation in making it happen—making you feel great about yourself and your relationship—seems to slip the minds of even the most ardent, contemporary, and insightful women.

Women's perceptions about their value as people are simultaneously affected by two primary arterial routes: how physically attractive they are and how much they're doing for others at home and at work. Being an active participant in satisfying sex is not a factor that has much weight when it comes to a positive self-image. We'll get to the part that looks play in self-image and sex in the next chapter, but right now our focus is on the other prong of the self-judgment fork—what they are doing for others.

Women working both inside and outside the home often feel the most pressure to produce, but this hardly exempts those who are stay-at-home moms. Contemporary housewives are incredibly busy. With today's excessive helicopter parenting being the norm and workout studios appearing everywhere, stay-at-home mothers are doing more than ever on behalf of their kids and figures. The top-notch mothers of today are the ones who do and think of everything for their children first, their figures second, others third, and their intimate partners last.

For nearly a decade, I was the director of sexuality counseling services at an exclusive wellness resort in Lenox, Massachusetts, that is a favored travel destination for affluent women between the ages of 25 and 70. Many of the guests would come for four days of rest and relaxation with gal pals. It is a great place to get away from the demands of kids, household management, and work and to reconnect with friends who are likely dealing with similar stressors. The irony was that these guests did very little resting or relaxing. What was supposed to be a kick-back-and-do-nothing weekend with friends would turn into an exercising, calorie-counting, four-day marathon topped off nightly with an expensive spa treatment they felt they deserved because they had been *so good* all day. After all, anyone who had exercised for six hours and only ate one air-filled merengue after a dinner totaling 250 calories was entitled to an expensive exfoliating treatment, right? The quid pro quo of these women's thinking—relaxation and pleasure can only be partaken of if you nearly kill yourself first—fascinated and saddened me. With rare exception, the women I saw for sexuality counseling who told me they loved their partners but had no interest in sex showed entirely too much interest in everything excluding their partners. What they did on behalf of their kids and their figures were top of the list when it came to measuring their self-worth. Unlike our own mothers, who didn't seem to mind a Danish with their coffee and adding more than a dash of "make the kids do it" to their parenting method, many modern women torture themselves with their diets and can't seem to get behind the idea that kids need chores. They fear that expecting them to do stuff and act responsibly will lower one of the following: their approval rating as mothers, their children's level of satisfaction in life, or their children's academic achievement. These are dangerous assumptions that can lead to incredible burnout for mothers as well as lazy kids who grow up always expecting someone else to do their work for them. Consider the following story told to me by one of the mothering escapees who came to see me with a complaint of a decreased libido. Although this is a bit extreme, it is a perfect example of just how overboard women can go when it comes to the responsibilities they unnecessarily assume.

> Before I left for this trip away, I created a Power-Point presentation for my husband and eleven-year-old daughter. I explained every aspect of household management I could think of so they would be prepared for any and all eventualities while I was away. I reviewed all the phone numbers they might need: the vet, pediatrician, grandparents, neighbors, and friends—you know . . . all that stuff. It also explained the meals I had prepared for them and how to heat them up. And, I listed nearby restaurants in case they decided to go out instead of eating at home. —*Beth, 39*

This story was the topper! I had never heard of someone going quite this far in her efforts to cover all bases. As part of my assessment and development of a strategy to help her realize how this was connected to her loss of interest in sex, I began by asking her two important questions: was her husband developmentally delayed, and did he and their daughter fight like cats and dogs? The answer to both questions: no. Her husband was the CEO of a major company and the two of them were crazy about one another. Both were looking forward to time alone together. I am certain that any CEO husband is more than likely to be able to manage for four days without his wife, especially while in the company of the apple of his eye. My guess: the two of them probably wouldn't eat anything she had prepared, would order their favorite takeout foods every night, or would eat candy the entire weekend and never have any reason to call folks on the help list—or 911. I couldn't help but laugh and feel deeply sympathetic; the obsessiveness and dedication to being in control of all things, at all times, was both comical and disturbing. It exemplifies what so many of my clients with low libidos do—entirely too much of what others could and should be doing for themselves, all in the name of feeling good about themselves. This kind of living not only interrupts the pursuit of pleasure, but also breeds resentment and terrible fatigue, neither of which lead to much pleasurable living or good sex.

When it's illuminated, smart women can see that their kids, partners, co-workers, and friends are able to take care of much of their own business and don't need their help to get the job done. But it's very difficult for them to say, "I can't help you with this" and believe that people will still like and love them. The dictate that doing for others at all costs is critical short-circuits your ability, from very early on in life, to develop hardwiring that attracts you to pleasure. In fact, most people don't ask two questions that are essential to living a pleasurable life: "What do I do every day that is pleasurable and sensual?" and "How do I keep my sensuality in the palm of my hand?" Without the answers to these questions in mind, we often make choices about coupling that don't add to our pleasure quotients. When it comes to choosing a long-term mate, we need to ask ourselves, "Is this person an intimate partner whose sexuality I truly enjoy, who I feel sexually satisfied with, who respects the importance of satisfying sex in our relationship, and who brings out the best in my sexuality?"

Women aren't trained to consider and integrate their feelings about pleasure and sexuality into their feelings about themselves as successful and satisfied people. As adults they end up doing things on their to-do lists in ways they feel are best and right, which results in an exaggerated sense of responsibility for having things done using very specific standards. Obsessive preoccupation with tasks being done correctly is really just a self-imposed mandate for women to complete the tasks themselves in order to ensure that they were done right. This is a common and dangerous pitfall that results in crippling fatigue and, predictably, shuts down libido.

THE STORY OF AN AVERAGE DAY

When 10 P.M. arrives, many women stare at the clock, thinking, *Oh my God, is it ten o'clock* already*?! How did this happen?* At this hour, working women and stay-at-home mothers are likely to have just woken up after their nap from bedtime reading, are just finishing the dinner dishes, or are crawling up the basement stairs with laundry that needs folding. When all is done to their satisfaction, they head to bed with immeasurable exhaustion and indescribable relief. *Ah, my pillow is only moments away!* What doesn't happen en route is a stop at the threshold of the boudoir to suddenly exclaim, "What was I *thinking*? Why was I wasting time loading the dishwasher, folding clothes, and applying moisturizer when we have a sex playpen in here? Come on, hot stuff! Let's put Hugh Hefner to shame." These weary, pleasure-starved, multitasking phenoms of home and office are so dog-tired they can barely see straight. They fall into their beds, grateful to be supine, and grab the best of women's "porn"—a novel, a catalog, or perhaps a magazine—laying on their bedside tables. Once in bed, the modern woman feels at rest, finally, and takes heart in no longer being on duty for anyone, at least for a while. Then, the unthinkable happens: she feels that all-too-familiar weight and heat and thinks, *Oh no, you've got to be kidding, right?* If the period of starvation has been long, the heat and weight start moving toward her like an inchworm and she hears those heartless, abhorrent words: "Honey, are you awake?" These four simple words are the worst words she could possibly hear from her mate after 10 P.M. Based on what women have told me, they'd rather hear just about anything else: "The house is on fire," "Mommy, I'm sick" (barf), or "Bad news, my cholesterol is 1,000." This marks an awful moment in time when women have to make a serious, painful decision: just how much can they afford to give to the charity of their choice, aka their loving relationship.

When I speak on the topic of women's sexual satisfaction, there are always audience members who say, "How did you know this? It sounds like you've been in my bedroom!" I know this because this is what women who have no libido tell me all the time. On first pass, they misconstrue the facts and blame their partners entirely: *What a greedy brute! Can't he/she see how much I do for our family and how tired I am? How much more am I supposed to give?* Plenty of women who come to see me with this complaint are convinced that their partners are the most selfish, oblivious people they've ever met. But these situations always form from contributions made by two people, not just one. While a woman may have a partner who loses sight of the demands of her day because of his or her own responsibilities, women can and do have their own blindspots and are quick to blame their partners for intruding on them in a way that really isn't intrusive at all. Tactless and poorly timed, probably. But intrusive is something completely different. Women's garden-variety disinterest in sex often goes hand in hand with a loss of pleasurable living and the self-empowerment that comes with it. A decreased libido is a common symptom that brings women in to see me for counseling. Once I pull the covers back on her bed-gone-cold, what lies beneath has little to do with sexuality and everything to do with choices she's made about how to live her life—as a multitasking, all-encompassing doer as opposed to a pleasure-seeking, do-what-you-can-and-keep-it-sane human woman. Taking on a steady diet of more than is necessary, safe, or sensible will leave you sleep deprived and upping the ante on what's needed to feel good about who you are. You can also count on it zapping your libido. The more you distance yourself from body-based pleasures and the powerful feelings they can give you, the less likely you are to refer to them for refueling when you're running on empty. This is why sex takes such a beating in so many marriages and in the lives of so many women who are wives and mothers.

Making Important Changes

Making the decision to become a parent is one of the most demanding and potentially rewarding things anyone can do. There is also a whacked-out aspect to it that you can neither prepare for nor comprehend ahead of time. I remember, early on in the life of my daughter, Thalia, walking down the hall at 3 A.M. wondering, *What on Earth was I thinking when I made the decision to get pregnant?* I felt an unprecedented, deep love in combination with a primal drive to meet her needs. But mixed in with this was physical exhaustion and shock over having given birth. The result: a strange state of mind insisting, *I must. I can't. I will, somehow* all at once. Fortunately for most babies and mothers, something magical happens to the majority of us when kids arrive on the scene. We manage to accommodate in ways that we never imagined possible.

In the beginning, when it comes to caring for our young, our impulses are not much different from those of a collie or calico. This is all good news. Then, as time goes by, our psychologies seep in and take over our thoughts and actions. Informed and sculpted by what we had and lacked as kids in our own families as well as cultural trends, we go on to develop a signature brand of child raising. This is where the absurd comes into play. It's remarkable to watch some of the crazy stuff women will do on behalf of their kids. And the conviction they have about it is even crazier. Woe be to the brave person who thinks he or she can gently and successfully guide women away from their strident and sometimes lunatic ideas of what's best for their kids. When most mothers set their minds to doing something they think is in the best interests of their children, just about nothing will dissuade them.

Experienced fathers and mothers alike—at least the honest ones—will admit that there was a phase of their child's life they found particularly obnoxious and difficult. This is hard to do until after your kids have passed into young adulthood and you've started counting all the many things you would do differently if you were given a second round with the same kids. But in general, we often hear from parents that the grade school years were the sweetest for them. Recollections of their children as primary school kids are often filled with dreamy, moist-eyed memories of school plays and picnics and storybook reading at bedtime that couldn't have been cozier or more satisfying. This couldn't have been further from the truth in my own life.

I found the decade when Thalia was in primary school to be one of the worst of my life, in part because I knew I was supposed to feel and act as though I loved every minute of it. As a full-time, full-scope midwife, I was seeing women in the office during the day and was up through the night with labor patients. This meant plenty of work outside the home, and inside it, too. There was clearly a case for my being tired, but I never felt that anyone was willing to talk about the tedium and drudgery of my home-based responsibilities: making lunches, doing laundry, civilizing kids, enforcing (and being limited by) regular bedtimes, listening to incessant uninteresting conversations, and arranging the almighty playdate. In fact, the attention being paid to virtually every little and big thing kids felt and did during these years was a big part of what nearly did me in, especially in combination with the demands of my work. Further, unless I made a specific plan to do something unrelated to mothering and kids that didn't involve my work, I would be trapped in the world of children and women who considered their children the most interesting and important things to talk about. Honestly, does everyone nowadays have gifted progeny with special dietary restrictions, a need for one-on-one attention at all times, and such delicate spirits that they could be broken irreparably by the slightest reprimand or off-color media exposure? The worst part about it was that I fell for this crap! I worked overtime to be one of those sensitive, all-knowing, all-giving mothers. Then finally, when my daughter was in fifth grade, I woke up and realized I'd better swoop in and do damage control double-time or she would end up being one of the biggest brats who ever lived and there would be nothing left of me.

I started my mothering rehabilitation program by re-signing as Thalia's laundress. She was ten. I did this when I realized she was putting her dirty laundry in a basket with clothes that I had already washed and folded for her. Her obliviousness irked me and forced me to face the facts: she didn't really care about my efforts with her wash and had grown very accustomed to having clean clothes appear from somewhere, ready for her to wear. I gave it serious thought and came to this conclusion: anyone who could figure out how to use the TV remote and a computer as easily as she had could certainly master the washer. I also decided it was time for her to gain an understanding of what it means to work for something you like and need—like clean clothes.

I continued my foray into the land of more old-fashioned parenting by paying less attention to everything she was doing and raising my expectations of her capacity to behave appropriately when faced with some of my needs. For example, when I was on call, I occasionally didn't have child care. This meant that she would have to come with me to the hospital while I was with someone in labor. She needed to sit at the nurses' station and color quietly or stay sequestered in the on-call room watching television. Whether she liked it or not was irrelevant. She did fine and it did her absolutely no harm. But, I paid dearly for this when I told a few people what my strategies were as a working midwife and head of household. I think they considered reporting me to Children's Protective Services for endangerment—as if exposing a child to the facts of life in real time were akin to having her on the set of a porn film. I also took a real beating from friends when I had my daughter, from ages six to eleven, fly on her own to visit my mother and sister for six weeks every summer.

People were shocked and very concerned that I would *let her go* and for *so long*. Somehow, they were either deaf or unable to process the fact that she was going to the Midwest to spend time with her grandmother and aunt, not John Wayne Gacy. My efforts to get a real break from daily mothering marked me as a parent under suspicion. People just couldn't accept that my parenting style was safe and might actually be in everyone's best interests. Because of it, Thalia gained confidence and independence, my relatives had her all to themselves, and I had a six-week reprieve from full-time mothering, which was great.

Fast-forward 16 years, and my now 22-year-old daughter is what I affectionately refer to as a "spin straw into gold" girl. She's been able to make many of her dreams come true because of the competence she's acquired. She is compassionate, has plenty of self-esteem, has direction in life, knows how to earn money by working hard, and is moving nicely toward being fully self-sufficient—all very important attributes. I am not saying that she never comes up with harebrained schemes or doesn't sometimes look to me as her financier for a poorly thought-out plan. But, in general, she's maturing nicely and gaining independence. I like to think this has something to do with the about-face I did as a parent. Maybe I'm wrong and I'm just lucky. But something tells me that the change in my expectations of her before she hit adolescence helped her become who she is as a young adult. The more I raised my expectations and my own awareness of the importance of my emotional health and sense of power in the world, the more mature and responsible she became and the better I felt about who I was in general and as a parent. In essence, I loosened my grip on everything in her world and got a firmer hold on things in my own.

The more I made an effort to realistically distinguish my choice of mothering responsibilities from Thalia's real needs as a kid, the more room and time I was able to make for things that were truly pleasurable and therefore beneficial to me. This was a deliberate, thoughtful, and regularly repeated endeavor on my part. Keeping this up depended on my making a concerted effort and giving it its due diligence. When I was honest about what my daughter needed me to do versus what I believed it was necessary for me to do, the list grew shorter on my end and longer on hers. I started to see that I had assumed responsibility for many things that she could and should do all by herself. This didn't always mean that her way of doing things matched mine; shoving stuff under her bed when asked to clean her room wasn't really what I had had in mind. But my objective of transferring more responsibility to her was to increase her awareness of the effort it took to meet her needs, give her more opportunities to accomplish this on her own, and loosen up more of my time and attachment to having things done a certain way. Eventually, it became a win-win for both of us: we both gained greater clarity about our individual responsibilities and self-respect for assuming them.

In addition to doing her laundry, spending summers with relatives, making her own lunches, and getting less attention from me, I also instituted the 4 or 6 x 36 rule for marital and sexual health and satisfaction. This meant that without fail, my partner and I went away every four to six weeks for a minimum of 36 hours. This gave us regular opportunities to escape and focus on bringing pleasure and sex back into our lives. My self-esteem and confidence soared after those weekends. Deliberately moving my identity as Thalia's mother aside for a chunk of time made room for other important parts of myself to surface—educated theatergoer, great conversational dinner date, and satisfying lover. Never mind mowing the lawn, putting on the screens, returning a breakfast invitation to friends, or doing whatever the kids might have had in mind for my weekend off. What I wanted and needed was to disappear with my partner, see an 11 A.M. matinee, have lunch at a new restaurant, and have sex in a fancy hotel in the afternoon. The strongest aphrodisiac of all is undivided attention, which we're only truly able to give when we love with integrity. In order to do this, we have to be fully present because we sincerely want to be. Loving anyone halfheartedly never has a good outcome. Think about it: if your partner admitted to you that he or she *mostly* loved you or loved you with *70 percent* of what they were worth, would this feel as though they were really in love with you? I doubt it. And in my experience, acting as if you're really in love when you're not will eventually take you down. Like a lion after an antelope on the African plains, your deceit will corner you, make your escape impossible, and then grab you by the throat, rip out your jugular, and eat you up. Loving without integrity is relationship treason and will erode the sovereign state of love and your markers of emotional well-being— eventually and unequivocally. I have heard and seen this in my practice a million times. If you're not fully in your relationship with your whole self, you'll feel bad about who you are. Taking time away from home to be alone with my partner allowed me the opportunity to give and receive undivided attention, to be reminded of the value of our loving and my sexuality. Without fail, this would reimmunize me against the invariably invasive negative thoughts I'd have about myself for reasons that really weren't substantive or meaningful. It also made me more able to deal with all sorts of things in life that didn't go my way.

I often work with women who haven't been away and alone with their partners for years, under the guise of responsible parenting. They try to convince me that this just wouldn't be in the best interests of their children. Consider this story from a woman who kept reassuring me about how much she loved her husband and was attracted to him, but simply had no interest in sex:

> I have been married to my husband for 15 years and we have three kids, ages 6, 9, and 13. I decided to leave my job to be home with our kids, which is really necessary because my husband travels so much for work. He is always asking me to meet him places that he goes to for business meetings. I have gone a couple of times since our kids were born, and it was great, but he doesn't seem to understand how hard it is for me to get away. Our kids really need me. They have organized activities, they really like me to be home, and I know they're not crazy about the people I have that could stay with them. I just feel I can't leave them. The few times I have gone with him, we have had great sex. I'm definitely attracted to him and I love him but, I can't have sex at home with our kids and all that's going on. And, I am exhausted by the end of every day. Sex is the last thing on my mind!
> —Arlene, 38

Red-light warning! This story is disturbing. None of these kids were nursing, no one had special needs, and this couple had the resources to hire someone to stay with their kids while they went away. Who cares if the kids didn't like the babysitter? As long as they're safe and reliable, then the kids just needed to find a way to cope with their dissatisfaction. This woman's decision to always stay behind is a setup for marital disaster and a sure formula for driving her libido underground forever and her mate into harrowing disappointment and anger. It also does nothing to expand or reinforce her sense of herself outside of mothering, or her experiences of pleasurable living and the power it grants her. If you can't afford to get away for a weekend, how about a long lunch and great afternoon sex in a local hotel once a month? Or, tell your kids you're off-duty at 8:30 once or twice a week and go to your room for time alone together. When they ask you what you're doing in there, tell them you need some romantic alone time. I guarantee they'll steer clear of your room while also getting the distinct message that loving relationships include time without kids around. Believe it or not, kids benefit from knowing that their parents want one another enough to still be intimate with each other. It's a comfort to know your parents' relationship is intact and purring. It transmits a message of security and stability that helps everybody relax.

Keep an Eye on Your Work

As the parent of a young adult who has recently graduated from college in a country whose economy has gone belly-up, I have my concerns about how exactly Thalia will be able to support herself. Despite my daughter's good work ethic, charming personality, and great looks, the fact is, she needs to make enough money to cover her expenses and still have some left over for life's pleasures. Given the high unemployment we've seen in the United States over the past five years, I worry that, after all her hard work in college, she'll have little opportunity to work in her field of study. In my discussions with her about "So, what's the plan?" she's always been quick to tell me that whatever work she does, it needs to be fun and she needs to enjoy

44

herself or she won't be doing it. This is an easy thing to say when you're 21 and don't have a family to support. However, Thalia makes an excellent point about the importance of enjoying what you do and keeping pleasure in your foreground while you're making enough money to live on.

Thalia's sensibilities about pleasure are sound and well integrated into her feelings of self-esteem and personal power. When she participates in things she enjoys and gets satisfaction from, she has a glow and vitality that is evident and sustaining. I can see this in her and have been able to actively track it; when she's been consumed by work, her vivaciousness wanes and she loses her enjoyment in and awareness of who she really is. When pleasure is tended to in the face of her responsibilities, the vitality that is all hers resurfaces. Her body and behavior are barometers of how closely she's sticking to her fundamental principles about living a pleasurable life.

Making decisions about work—staying in a job, leaving it, choosing it in the first place—are complicated ones that most of us will need to make more than once throughout our adult lives. Once we land jobs that pay well, especially in our fields, we're reticent to give them up just because we don't like them anymore. Having to evaluate my own pleasure in a job I had thrived in for almost a decade was something I personally faced a couple of years ago. I had wonderful colleagues whom I adored and who loved and supported me and my work, but I had reached the glass ceiling and the opportunities for continued growth and enjoyment were virtually nonexistent. I felt as though I was living in a skipping record—the same track playing over and over again—and I was so unhappy. I made the decision to leave when I finally realized that the impact of my lack of pleasure in my work life was corroding my pleasurable living outside of work also. I had fallen into a pit of asen-sual, robotic living that had me driving to work like an au-tomaton, doing my job with almost no finesse, and then coming home at the end of the day with nothing left for myself or my partner. I felt bad about myself, my ability to find anything pleasurable had waned, and my interest in sex had disappeared. In retrospect, I realize that I have never had less sex in my marriage than I did during the year I was making the decision to leave my longtime, fancy job. Colleagues desperately wanted me to stay on and even continued their campaigning after I left. They missed me and the status quo hadn't been that bad, right? Wrong. The work wasn't pleasurable anymore. I couldn't stand the administration, I dreaded my daily responsibilities, and ev-erything looked and felt flat to me. I wanted to feel good again about what I was doing in my professional life. I never told my colleagues that my sex life was suffering as a re-sult of hating my work and workplace, but this was true. This made my work as a sexuality counselor difficult to do with any sense of integrity and it was wearing on me, as it should have. If my own sexual energy is nowhere to be found, I am incapable of helping others when their sexual lives are faltering.

Choosing a job or leaving one because you feel it may be in the best interests of your sexuality may seem crazy, but it affects the whole of your sense of power and emo-tional well-being in the long run. I understand and can support people's decisions to take something on for the short term when the money is great or the position will boost your résumé in ways that you can't turn down. The problem is that too many of us don't make these choices with a short-term plan in mind. Once we're there, we're reticent to leave, even when we can feel the deleterious effects that our choice is having on everything else that's pleasurable in our lives and, most important, our feelings about ourselves. By the time I left my job, I was emotionally exhausted and in that terrible, dark place where you question your intuition—even though I knew I had made the right choice in leaving. When your work is plaguing you and draining all your energy for anything pleasurable, including sex, it's highly likely that your self-esteem is dwindling too. As much as I wanted to please my longtime, beloved colleagues, staying in my job would have been lethal and taken all the joy out of my life.

A strong work ethic is an important thing to have and something worth instilling in our kids but never at the expense of mental and physical health. Better to live on a smaller (or even very tight) budget than to lose your emotional health by pimping yourself for a bigger paycheck.

LOVING YOUR WORK BUT DOING TOO MUCH OF IT

But what if you love your work? It's creative. It makes you feel good about yourself. You can handle the ups and downs. This is a fabulous thing in life—and also a dreadful trap. This can be true for women and men, but we gals have a harder time coming back to pleasure and staying sexually afloat without the chemical magic of plenty of testosterone. Men's higher testosterone levels frequently remind them of how great sex is, even when they're supposed to be thinking about things decidedly not sexual (some people have all the luck). In combination with women's learned ability to put their figures and efforts on behalf of others first and sex on the back burner, loving your work and being good at it is likely the biggest trap you'll face when it comes to losing your libido. You'll just be sitting there, day in and day out, loving yourself for what you do on the job and forgetting about what you do—or aren't doing—in bed.

If you're a woman who has struck pay dirt at work, keep in mind that no matter how much your workplace appreciates you, they're unlikely to close up shop if you're hit by a truck; your partner, on the other hand, is another story. Think of it this way: if you have the good fortune of knowing well in advance that the Grim Reaper is coming to visit you and you're holding your beloved's hand in preparation for death, what parting words would you prefer to utter: "Gee, I wish I had put in more hours on the job" or "I am so glad I never let my work life get in the way of our life"? Neither the job itself nor your doing the work could ever be more important than your loving partnership and the sexuality between you—that is, if you honestly feel this way. If not, then put this book down, throw it in the trash, or pass it along to a friend. Unless you invented fire, you're just not as important in your workplace as you might be thinking you are. The smoldering embers you tend with your partner are far more important than the three-alarm fires you're always putting out at work.

The experience of actually setting limits in the workplace is daunting for most women. Imagining yourself saying something like "Thank you for having such confidence in me, but I am afraid I cannot take this on" feels like having a big fish bone caught in your throat and not knowing what to do. Move one muscle and it might get lodged there and cut off your windpipe. If you don't die by choking, your feelings of being ungenerous to your boss or colleagues will haunt you. And, whether or not what's being requested of you makes sense is irrelevant. I hear it all the time: "I can't believe they asked me to take this on—are they crazy?" "This isn't right and it's not even what I do, but . . . I can't say no." "It's too risky and I really don't want to manage the fallout from saying no." Buck up, girlie, and go back and review the tenets of the feminist movement. The idea behind women's liberation is not that women are supposed to do everything simultaneously. The issue is choice, and therefore having the right to choose what you want to do and are really able to do and when. Being fully vested in the workforce and having a family doesn't mean allowing your work in the office and at home to consume you or gobble up every ounce of energy you have for living a pleasurable life. If your self-esteem is dependent on your job performance and especially if people in your life tell you you've taken on too much, pay attention to what they're saying and remember that *no one* is irreplaceable in their job. If you're *always* so tired that you can't bring any pleasure into your life, then it's time to rethink what you've chosen to do. As difficult as this might be to do, the longer you live in a world of overwork (as an employee and/or mother) the more you'll acclimate to it and then you're sure to be like the frog in the pot that doesn't notice how hot the water has gotten until it reaches the boiling point. Take charge of what's happening—delegate tasks to responsible people, learn to work smart instead of hard, and keep things in perspective. Remember, your work world won't stop in its orbit if you die, but your loving partner's will.

QUESTIONS TO ASK YOURSELF

1. What is my self-esteem dependent on?

2.   Could I imagine life without a to-do list? If not, why?

3.   What are three tasks that I know my children are capable of doing on their own but I have continued to assume responsibility for? Why won't or can't I insist they do these things themselves?

4.   On a scale of one to ten, with one being the least and ten being the most, how much do I need to be in control of tasks and to have them done my way because it's the only right way?

5.   Do my work responsibilities take over my life on a frequent basis and interfere with my time with and energy for my partner?

6.   What would really happen if I set more limits on my availability to my children and to my job? What would the fallout be? What benefits might there be?

CHAPTER 3

I'M TOO FAT TO HAVE SEX

*I've been on a constant diet for the last two decades.
I've lost a total of 789 pounds. By all accounts, I should
be hanging from a charm bracelet.*

—ERMA BOMBECK

I have been taking care of women of all ages for over 20 years, and I am certain that I can count on one hand the number of women who have told me they like their bodies. The complaints and criticisms that women have about their figures and its particulars are endless. This is true whether they've acquired a shape through no fault of their own or as the result of eating and exercise patterns that don't promote health. Women's litanies are far-reaching and can be absolutely ludicrous: my ass is too flat; my breasts are too large or too small (and of course, thanks to gravity, all our breasts sag sooner or later); I wish I had blue eyes, not brown; I'm all hips; my upper arms waddle. Women loathe their hair, the shapes of their faces, their complexions, and they just can't stand their legs. The list goes on and on. But, the most predictable and consistent complaint women have about their bodies has to do with fat—its distribution, the overall amount, and its reportedly unrelenting presence, no matter what one does. Ironically, this is true for many women regardless of how much they actually weigh, their overall fitness level, or how old they are.

On last count, there were approximately 2,222,222,222 books on the market written specifically for women who are looking to slim down, beef up, or beautify. So, why do so many of us either find it difficult to follow the advice of the "experts" or still hate ourselves even when we do and bear visible evidence of that? Evidently, making friends with our flesh—no matter how much of it we really have in whatever locations—is one of the most arduous, consuming, expensive, and emotionally upsetting accomplishments women attempt throughout life. Even Eve Ensler, the feminist activist and author of *The Vagina Monlogues,* who advocates for women to be accepted and respected for exactly who they are, has felt the pain of body hatred. In her book *The Good Body,* she writes: "What I can't believe is that someone like me, a radical feminist for nearly thirty years, could spend this much time thinking about my stomach. It has become my tormentor, my distractor: it's my most serious committed relationship. It has protruded through my clothes, my confidence, and my ability to work. I've tried to sedate it, educate it, embrace it, and most of all, erase it."[3] The idea that her ongoing hatred for her stomach represented her "most serious committed relationship" left me speechless.

I personally have had an above-average fat quotient since the age of two. Long before the United States was tackling an epidemic of pediatric obesity, I was sitting front and center as the poster child for what could happen if a kid really loved to eat and was genetically coded to be full figured rather than slim no matter what. Despite the endless hours I spent on my bike and playing sports and my genuine enjoyment of exercise from an early age, none of my regular and vigorous physical activity seemed to make a difference when it came to my essential tendency to store calories versus shedding them. I was destined to be a woman with an ample figure. The genes of my petite Greek mother and strapping Czechoslovakian father came together to create a broad-shouldered, buxom, farm-animal-strong girl whose only noticeably Greek feature are her eyes—those are from Asia Minor and are the only things that reflect my Mediterranean heritage. Everything else about how I look comes from my father's side of the family, and they were all big people. I, like everyone else, came into the world with my genetics predetermined. But genetics aren't everything, and we all have control over how we behaviorally and psychologically manage what nature has bestowed upon us from birth.

As kids, my sister and I spoke Greek first and English second, which gave us both a tremendous advantage when it came to the authenticity of our accents. When I lived in Greece for several months in my early 20s, most Greeks—on first pass—assumed I was German until I began speaking and sounded just like they did. Once we cleared the hurdles of language and confirmation of my Greek roots, all the Greeks I met—true to their outspoken natures—were perfectly comfortable asking me how I got to be so big. I have to admit, the story of Gulliver and the Lilliputians would cross my mind often since just about everyone in the country seemed smaller than I was. But in truth, I am not a giant nor have I allowed myself to become a candidate for the job of fat lady in the circus. I am a robust woman who wears a women's size 16 or 18—unquestionably making me a plus-size shopper. However, and most important, I don't consider my size to be the core of my identity. This is not true for many of the women I have worked with as a sexuality counselor, especially women who seek me out as a result of a lack of interest in sex.

Unfortunately, the seeds of self-hatred concerning body image are planted early in life when the virtues of beauty and grace are extolled. The messages girls get are that slim and pretty are one and the same, that any kind of sexiness exhibited runs the risk of being seen as slutty, and that no matter what, you're best off if you turn away from your sexuality and focus your attentions elsewhere.

Then in adolescence, when our sexuality comes knocking with force and persistence, the risk of self-loathing is doubled if we get the message that keeping our high standing as good girls also means turning a deaf ear to our longings and desires to look sexy and be sexual with another person. The feedback and education many girls get about their sexuality and desire to experiment with sex in their appearance and actions is terrifying and deterring: they're told to look pretty and slim but *not* sexy and that if they have sex they *will* get pregnant, contract a disease, or ruin their reputations. In American culture, the concept that having satisfying and responsible sex could actually enhance a teen girl's self-esteem is blasphemous and bizarre. Girls grow up needing to hide their sexual feelings and forays, which eventually results in pushing sex as far to the periphery as possible. They learn that it's better, safer, and more universally acceptable to just stick with their efforts to stay slim and attractive.

Sadly, following this party line not only creates an environment that is devoid of pleasure, it also sets up the view that physical appearance is the most important part of attractiveness. It is a sad but common story.

Women who fall victim to this idea often use their weight as their primary self-identifying feature. They have lost perspective on themselves as unique individuals and their appeal as whole people. Their preoccupation with physical beauty—as opposed to physical or mental health—distorts their perceptions of who they are and how the rest of the world feels about them. Being overweight makes many women feel undeserving of pleasure, like it is something that must be earned. They believe that the more flesh you have, the less pleasure you're entitled to. Women in these straits have lost their ability to feel or see—literally and figuratively—what's real about their bodies and what isn't. They also become selectively deaf to any positive comments they receive about how appealing and desirable they are. This makes the possibility of sexual intimacy with a loving partner (or even yourself) extraordinarily complicated if not impossible.

FAT AND SEX ARE NOT MUTUALLY EXCLUSIVE

Throughout my years of caring for women, especially in the context of sexuality counseling, I have sat for countless hours with women who tell me their fat and their feelings about it are the sole reasons they are estranged from feeling sexy and having sex. Despite the mournful calls of their desperately lonely and hungry partners who desire them, if a woman thinks of herself—primarily—as overweight, she'll likely spurn his or her overtures and do all she can to avoid physical and sexual intimacy. Her partner's opinion of her body is irrelevant. In fact, sometimes a partner's acceptance of and pleasure in her physical being will leave her suspicious of their sincerity or can even fuel her fire of self-hatred. This counterintuitive outcome only creates further complications, including tremendous resentment between the couple. The bottom line is the woman's opinion of herself. In the absence of any positive feelings about her appearance or even positive regard for what her body can allow her to experience, a woman can lose her sexuality in a millisecond and have to struggle mightily to retrieve it.

The following stories told to me by women in my practice illustrate what I am talking about. Although initially they may not appear to share a common theme, the connection between all three will become evident.

> I have been married to my husband for 16 years and would describe the marriage as essentially good. But unfortunately, we haven't been very sexually active over the last three years. My interest in sex waned considerably after our third child was born, and I attribute this mostly to the fatigue from working and parenting but also to the fact that I don't look good anymore. I gained weight with each pregnancy and haven't been able to lose it. By the time my third baby was born, I was a lot heavier, and this really bothered me. I have tried losing weight but haven't been successful, and I'm discouraged about how my figure has changed and the potential impact that being heavier could have on my health. It has also become an issue for my husband. He has broached the subject, saying that he was concerned about my health, but then he added that he missed my "other

body" sometimes. This really hurt. He did say that he's not expecting me to look the way I did when we were first married, but he said that he doesn't really feel like I look like my real self anymore. The combination of the added weight and my decreased fitness and health is less appealing to him. He bought me a gym membership, has offered to watch the children anytime I want to exercise, and is even willing to help with cooking healthy meals at home. But, once I really knew how he felt about how I look, sex was really out of the question for me. He says he wants to have sex with me, but then he tells me that he wants me to be thinner. So which is it, and what can I really believe is sincere? —Elizabeth, 44

I'm 55 and while I stopped having a period a couple of years ago, I still have occasional hot flashes, I don't sleep well, and my vaginal dryness makes having sex really uncomfortable. Other than these menopause problems, the only health issue I have is high blood pressure, which runs in my family. I take medicine for it and am doing fine, so I'm not worried about that. The other thing menopause did is give me this belly fat, and I hate it. It's *so* hard to lose any weight. I feel like my body is just disgusting! It's really intolerable for me. My partner, Karen, and I have been together for over 20 years and we're close in age, but she doesn't seem to be having menopause problems to the same extent as I am. She also hasn't lost her interest in sex and, even though I can't stand my body, she still tells me she wants me and doesn't feel the same way about my body as I do. Actually, the fact that we're not having sex is a real problem for her. I am depressed about the changes in my body, and I feel really hopeless about aging and can't find anything positive to say about myself. I know that I'm lucky to have pretty good health. But when I come home from work, I am so tired and so unhappy that I am finding

myself drinking more wine and zoning out with the tele-vision. I am hoping that there is some kind of hormonal treatment that you can give me that will help me with the weight loss and the dryness, and maybe you have something that will help with my sex drive, too. I have to do something. I have to find a way to have sex again.
—*Barbara, 55*

I've always been a large woman—always about 250 pounds. My husband tells me how beautiful I am and that he likes my body, that my weight isn't a problem for him. While I always enjoyed sex in the past, something has changed. On the one hand, I am thrilled that I have a husband who thinks I am pretty and doesn't torture me about my weight. But, I am not comfortable or happy about how heavy I am anymore. Plus I'm worried about developing diabetes. This has ended up affecting our sex life. I just don't want to have sex until I lose some weight. I just can't reconcile with my husband's accep-tance of my body when I am trying so hard to change it! No matter what my partner says to me, I can't seem to set aside my bad feelings and enjoy sex with him the way I used to. I finally told him I just couldn't have sex with him until I lost weight and this really upset him. I feel like no matter which way I go, I can't win: I don't feel like I can have sex until I am thinner and I am disappoint-ing my husband by doing this. I don't know how long it will take me to lose the weight I want to, but this isn't really working for us the way things are now. —*Carol, 37*

As a sexuality counselor and midwife, I always use a combination of sympathy and compassion, speaking the truth, and helping women reestablish their priorities to help guide them out of their suffering. Whether I am about to deliver their baby, help them manage with the normal discomforts of menopause, or help them find their way out of a sexual conundrum, I don't hesitate to give advice based on logic, fact, and common sense. It's always my intention to help people manage the seemingly unmanageable with information and strategies that are within their capabilities. In order to do this they need to be reacquainted with the facts of their situation and confronted head-on with their negative and false thinking.

Elizabeth was struggling with an odd combination of problems: simple inertia, an unwillingness to be completely truthful with herself, and a persistent tendency to blame her partner for their sexual problems. Both she and her husband acknowledged that her weight was a problem and that it was impacting their sex life and possibly her health. However, Elizabeth blamed her husband for his "rejection" and wasn't doing anything to create the change they both desired. Somehow, her lack of success in losing weight and becoming more physically fit got twisted into a scenario that described her husband as rejecting her as a sex partner because of her fat. She had de-emphasized her own feelings when reciting the story, creating a tale of villain versus victim that just wasn't true. Elizabeth's husband hadn't called her terrible names, shamed her, or said he wouldn't have sex with her until she lost weight. Instead, he had given a kind voice to what they both were feeling: her weight had become a problem that had gone unaddressed for too long. He was being honest and attempting to be supportive of her making a change they would both welcome with an outcome they mutually agreed would be in her best interests.

Barbara's vaginal dryness, continuing hot flashes, and belly fat may have felt like her most upsetting menopausal symptoms, but frankly, these were the least of her problems.

Barbara's upset and negative feelings about her body were being managed—unsuccessfully—with increased alcohol consumption. She was on a slippery slope headed toward disaster where this was concerned. Unfortunately, her story is a very common one. I work with many midlife (and younger) women whose glass of red or white at the end of a hard day becomes their best friend. Unbeknownst to them, the more alcohol they drink, the higher their risks are for continued hot flashes, sleep disruption, weight gain, and preventable health problems. And, I have yet to meet someone who becomes inebriated on a nightly basis and doesn't fall prey to inertia about plenty of things, including sex with their partner. This is a vicious cycle: the more you drink, the more depressed you become because of your inability to make changes, then you drink more to anesthetize yourself against the upset over your inertia. I could relieve Barbara's vaginal dryness with topical estrogen and help her develop healthier exercise and eating habits. However, she needed to be consistently sober to take my suggestions. The good news was that she *was* aging and *had* a loving partner—after all, her alternative at 55 would be what most of us would consider a premature death and a life without love. Essentially, her health was good. But, she was slowly ruining it by drinking too much and living with a negative attitude about herself as an aging woman. Given that her only health problem was mild hypertension, she was really doing better than she realized. But in her mind, her body was betraying her. She felt disempowered, her pleasure quotient had hit rock-bottom, and sex felt like an impossibility.

Carol's desire to lose weight and improve her fitness was healthy, and it deserved recognition and support. But, her idea that she couldn't be sexual until this happened was unreasonable—to both herself and her partner. The idea that sex would be her reward when (and if) she reached her goals was robbing her of pleasure that could potentially support and encourage her in her efforts to lose weight and improve her health. The belief that fat people don't deserve pleasure or sex is common, and it fuels the negative attitudes so many of us have about our bodies.

FINDING YOUR WAY OUT OF THE WEB

The first order of business for all women dealing with challenges like these is to work through the emotions associated with them. Step one: face the fact that women of all shapes and sizes have and deserve pleasure and sex. The body you don't think deserves to have sex because it's so fat is the same body you allow to enjoy other things without restriction based on poundage—like hugging people you love, listening to music, petting your dog, and shopping for new shoes. Most important, when your partner is telling you he or she loves your body, that it feels like home to them, and that they want you, why do you call their longing a lie and an impossibility? Would you do this to them about anything else that brings them comfort and pleasure? I doubt it. In fact, you'd probably encourage their partaking of these other things and take great pleasure in the comfort they bring them. So what happens when their object of desire and comfort is you?

You also need to step back and try to look at the situation without clouding your judgment with negative opinions about weight. Elizabeth, who wasn't successful in making changes to her figure; Barbara, who had unrealistic expectations about aging and drank to excess; and Carol, who was unhappy with her weight, all had essentially accepting, loving, and supportive partners. They had lovers who were attracted to them and wanted them to live long and healthy lives—and this is the case in the majority of the relationships I see.

So what is it that brings on this self-hatred and low self-esteem? Often, it's a negative mantra you repeat, telling yourself that you can't have sex because of your shape and size. If you're plagued by an internal dialogue such as this, I suggest you play a game of hot potato—whenever the negative thoughts come into your head imagine them as hot potatoes that you have just caught unawares. When a hot potato comes into your hands, you drop it to avoid getting burned. We can work with negative thoughts in this same way. This is hard to do at first. But, with persistence and practice, dropping the negative thoughts gets easier. I learned this technique at a meditation retreat once and find it very helpful. When I start my own roll of negative thoughts about my body, I let them come in and then drop them as quickly as I can. I then do my best to replace them with something else while also getting up and moving—which is an effective way to change my experience of my body.

In addition to working to change your thinking by dropping negative thoughts, realize that your effort to do so is a very sexy thing. This is rarely considered or talked about. When you love someone who has a problem they're working hard to change for the better, it's got a lot of appeal. There is something that happens to our entire person when we put forth sincere effort to make changes to improve our lot in life. We become the ultimate cool cats when we commit ourselves to self-empowering change, and our ranking on the sexy meter soars. We can feel it, and that's all it takes to start the ball rolling. Once we feel this way about ourselves, others notice and it's all good from that point onward.

Elizabeth was blaming her husband for feeling the same way about her extra weight as she did and was holding out. Barbara was attempting to drink away her sadness about aging and not discussing it openly with her partner—and she was refusing to have sex because of it. Carol, who would likely have gotten lots of calls if she had been on the Big Beautiful Babes dating website, had decided to strike against the guy who wanted her no matter what. I helped these women see the true situations they were in—which had some real pluses—and in so doing hoped to reduce the sting of their psychic burn of self-loathing. This isn't a cure for all negative thinking. It's a coping mechanism for when pervasive negative thoughts persist, and it's important for you to do this if you're working your way through similar problems. Now, let's move on to some tactics and strategies that can have immediate results in your ability to bring pleasure and sex back into your life.

Physical Tactics and Strategies

So here we go: the most important thing is to move first, then eat—and laugh while you're doing both.

When women hate their bodies, I always recommend that their first step toward reuniting with pleasure be regular and frequent movement: yoga, dancing, walking, bicycle riding, and, swimming. Any single activity or combination of several is the place to begin. Think about how bad you feel when your movement is restricted or limited for some reason; this will help motivate you in the direction you need to go. Movement is an important first step to living fully in your body, which is an absolute prerequisite for feeling powerful, accessing pleasure, and experiencing satisfying sex.

No doubt you're thinking, *Oh, here we go again. It's the exercise prescription, of course. This book isn't saying anything we haven't heard before.* Yes and no.

Moving in as many different ways as you're able to will keep you capable of enjoying your body as much as possible for as long as possible, which is the first step to being willing to share it with someone in an intimate way. And all those books out there that talk about exercise for fitness rarely say a peep about improving your access to pleasure or satisfying sex. My focus and the words I use are different and can spin your perspective toward health, pleasure, powerful living, and sexual satisfaction and away from a focus on weight loss. Moving more, expanding your range of motion, decreasing body pain, increasing fitness and stamina, and reducing your risks of ill health are what I am after. If weight loss occurs as a consequence, so be it. An expanded range of motion, greater fitness, and less body pain will lead to your having more personal power to do the things you want to do. You'll have greater self-esteem, confidence, and pleasure. A frequent and welcome consequence of all three is an increased interest in sex.

Most women I work with who are struggling with their body images have an unhealthy relationship with movement; either they never get off the sofa or they're exercise addicts. Neither of these is healthy or safe. Personally, if my interest in pleasure and sex has waned, I first do an assessment of how physically active I've been in the preceding month to see whether I have fallen off my curve. I enjoy swimming, walking, riding my bicycle, and a little bit of yoga stretching, and I love to dance. These are the physical activities that best suit me and that I really enjoy. Human beings are not bumps on logs, nor do we have the hard wiring to move all the time like Australian shepherds do. Both moving too little and too much can distance you from the real pleasure to be had in moving sensibly for your age, body type, and health.

If a woman is really serious about improving her sex life, she'll be willing to let go of some of her purely cerebral undertakings or change her commitment to participating in the Ironman competition so she can enjoy physical activity in a more commonsense and sustainable way. The underlying principle that I emphasize when it comes to moving is to move primarily for the pleasure of it. Moving is a meditation, a time for reflection and relaxation. It helps with pain relief, improves sleep, and is the best thing ever for your heart. This is a very different way to look at exercise than we're accustomed to, and it's far more appealing than counting reps and miles and putting your original set of joints at risk from overuse.

When I talk with women about this, frequent first responses include the following: "I'm too embarrassed to exercise," "I don't have time!" and my favorite, "I am not very good at anything physical." I am by no means a good Middle Eastern dancer, but I love the music and have managed to reconcile with the fact that my belly fat can move in one direction while my best intentions move in another. I just pretend it's not happening and remain on the lookout for just the right skirt to conceal this unfortunate fact while staying within the fashion of the genre. Unlike Samia Gamal—who danced in the 1954 film *Ali Baba and the Forty Thieves*—I know I will not be approached by any film producers. But, I don't let this interfere with my enjoyment or imagination when I dance along to the *baladi* rhythms.

This music reminds me of my childhood and the dancers in the clubs that we went to as a family. This is where I was first introduced to the art of belly dancing, which I have revered and enjoyed since I was a little girl. One benefit of those excursions with my vociferous relatives and their friends at neighboring tables was the frequent comments (all in Greek, of course, which is always loud and impassioned) about just how beautiful the rolls, curves, and full bosoms of the dancers were. It was a festival of appreciation of the flesh and a great foundation for me. And heaven help the dancer if she was too thin. That meant disparaging comments and fewer bills of lower denominations made their way into her coin belt. Granted, it was just the right amount of flesh necessary to pique the interest of the audience members. But, it was the enthusiasm of my family over the fleshiness in and of itself that infused me with the confidence I needed at 52 to walk into the dance studio and say to Carmen, "Teach me all you can." I wouldn't have missed out on that experience for anything.

Belly dancing may not be your thing, and that's fine. But we all have something we like to do with our bodies. Or, perhaps, want to do but have never found a way to do it well or safely. Give some thought to what you used to do as a kid or fantasies you've had as an adult. You'd be surprised by the good that can come from your fantasies if you just let them come to life, even if your real-life version isn't exactly what your fantasy is. Let go of whatever restrictions you've placed on yourself because of fear, embarrassment, or lack of instruction or time and devise ways to participate in the essential activity. For instance, I love to ride my bike. I wish I could be one of those lean demons effortlessly pushing themselves up hills all over my rural community, but this goes beyond my capacity and comfort zone. So, I ride my bike on flat bike paths and enjoy it nonetheless. Make an effort to resurrect or create what you want to do and see what comes of it. I guarantee, the more you move, the more powerful you'll feel, the more pleasure you'll experience, and the more you'll like who you are.

What about Food and Eating?

So, let's say you are a woman who is undeniably fat. Or, you've been fighting excess calorie consumption your whole life and if you don't pay very close attention, you will be undeniably fat—even *very fat*—in short order. Either way, we all know we win some battles and we lose others. I have days when I simply can't explain how I ate an entire box of vanilla sandwich creams. I don't know how it happens. Other days, my diet is exemplary, demonstrating impressive self-control and sensibility. Those of you who experience these extravaganzas of consumption are easily convinced that there's an inverse relationship between how much you're eating and the amount of pleasure you're allowed; after all, your crime should be punishable somehow. Let's face it, after you've consumed a week's worth of calories during one car ride, your focus is more on moving from behind the steering wheel than doing anything pleasurable with your body. In fact, if there were stocks in front of you once you got out of the car, all the better. You could put yourself in them and start your penance immediately. If you're someone who faces this vexing and disdain-inducing experience often, I recommend you consult with an expert for advice—so, here I go.

I, like many of my clients, have lived in and through various degrees of fatness throughout my life. However, I have remained open to pleasure and have always enjoyed sex, no matter how much I have weighed. I also have always had relatively nonoverweight partners and, in fact, have never been intimate with a person of my own size, regardless of the state of largeness I happened to be in. Believe it or not, I can actually attribute some of this good fortune to my mother.

I grew up with a mother who convinced me that my weight and naturally large body should never be an impediment in pursuing something or achieving what I really wanted in life—except wearing a bikini or miniskirt. These two clothing items were not acceptable attire for someone who had a figure like mine. But, everything else I wanted was fine and should have nothing to do with how much I weighed. I am sure at the time she wasn't thinking that her emotional support and non-fat-hating opinions would positively influence my sexuality but lucky for me, they did. My mother's beliefs were not influenced or swayed by her own body size, which has never gone beyond a women's petite size 10. Either because her love for me was blindingly powerful or because my little mother loved a large man herself, her opinions of what was attractive were broad and atypical and seem to have immunized me against a degree or specific kind of self-hatred that could have eaten away at my self-esteem and experiences of pleasure my entire life. Instead, what happened was that I developed a kind of self-deprecating humor that has served me well and an approach to food and eating that I fine-tune over and over again but generally don't feel overcome by. Have I ever considered drastic measures like bariatric surgery or starvation diets? Of course I have. Anyone who is even slightly overweight considers those things, and if they tell you otherwise, they're lying. But, the fact is, I am rather physically fit and do not subscribe to the surgery-can-fix-anything model. The real key to managing my occasional and intermittent self-loathing about my weight is to mastermind my own insurrection against my darkest thoughts.

In the case of my big body, I decided that the real problem was not that my bigness itself was an impediment to what I wanted in life—minus the bikini. The real problem I faced when it came to food was my frequent tendency to look to it for comfort and information. I was repeatedly mistaking those vanilla sandwich creams for a brilliant psychiatrist, best friend, great comedy, or flawless partner. This never works! No matter how many cookies I ate, I was never rewarded with oracular insight, nor did I feel I had the answer to all things. In fact, it was quite the opposite. Eventually, I came to terms with the fact that cookies have an IQ of zero. I also finally admitted (in the privacy of my own mind) that every time I ate a million of them, I didn't become more adept at problem solving—just uncomfortably full and incapable of conceiving of myself as a sexually active human. Eventually, by reminding myself of this *repeatedly,* and in combination with my genuine love of moving, my body shrank by 50 pounds or so, which has stayed off for several years now. No magic pills, no fancy diets, no surgery. Things changed when I sat alone and thought about what the cookies and all other baked goods worldwide had the true potential of providing for me: *many* delicious, nutrient-empty calories and no improved insight into anything. While all this metamorphosis was occurring, I continued to have great sex and find ways to make fun of the struggle I faced every day to establish a more reasonable relationship with the things I loved to eat. And, I am *still* working on this—and I'm guessing that will be the case for the rest of my life.

What's hardest for many of us who eat way too much food is changing our minds and developing a lasting belief that if we eat less we won't be missing out on something fantastic. We also have to shed the bizarre notion that at any moment we might be facing our very own version of the Last Supper and, therefore, need to eat as much as we can—just in case.

If you want to change your eating habits, you have to decide what your rules and opinions are about food: what you can and can't live without, what you can do to eat less food, and whether you believe that eating less means you'll be healthier and more comfortable. Let's be honest, none of us likes to feel stuffed after having eaten too much, and all of us enjoy the sensation of genuine hunger. Feeling hungry makes me feel like a paragon of virtue. It also gives me a legitimate reason to eat. Imagine having this feeling every day—even more than once a day. This is a great fantasy that can actually come true for nearly everyone.

My rules include the following: I try very hard not to eat after 7 P.M., I only eat dessert on Sundays and Wednesdays, I eat very little butter, I rarely drink alcohol or soda, and I avoid trance eating by not eating in my car unless I have no choice. I also eat three meals each day and avoid snacking. And, I reserve the vanilla sandwich creams for one of the two days of the week when I allow dessert to cross my lips. This is what works best for me the majority of the time. But to be truthful, I mess up on this with some frequency. And I even continue to mistake vanilla sandwich creams for the Magic 8 Ball, which we all know has *all* the answers. I can't deny that the enjoyment I experience from the flavors and textures of my favorite foods leads me astray. And now, at 53, I am facing the facts of aging and how this is affecting my figure and my health. But I do all I can to stay on track, and when I veer off course or have a bad food day or week I do my best to get back on track and remind myself—yet again—of the zero IQ of all foods. I also weigh myself a couple of times a week. It keeps me honest and conscious of how my eating and moving are affecting my weight. And, I keep moving as much and as often as possible.

We all have foods we like—or look to for guidance— that, in all honesty, we can imagine ourselves living without. Review your eating habits and food choices. Unless you've been living under a rock, you've had enough exposure to know what's causing your extra poundage and what would be in your best interests to eliminate. And if you're really stumped about this, let your body do the talking and give it the respect it deserves by listening. How do you feel after you've downed a couple of doughnuts? Dandy or disgusted? Are you reciting Shakespeare by heart after your second glass of Malbec or slurring your words like a fool? How about your waistband? Has it gotten tighter after going to three birthday parties and consuming too much cake? I am not asking that you disclose your food crimes in the public square at high noon. But, I am highly recommending that you acknowledge them to yourself. Then, read food labels, increase your consciousness about how and what you eat, and make the changes *you* can live with to improve your relationship with food instead of being imprisoned and poisoned by it. If you can't do this alone, go to a local chapter of Overeaters Anonymous, find a good counselor, or keep a food diary—or maybe all of the above.

You may be a woman who would benefit from talking with a health care provider who is skilled and interested in helping patients establish healthy eating and exercise habits. This conversation doesn't happen often enough in the exam rooms of American practitioners. My colleagues don't have time, and they often don't know what to say to their patients. They also don't necessarily have healthy lifestyles themselves, making it more difficult to discuss one with you. They may also simply not be able to identify with your struggle, which you'll detect and which will make it an even less successful conversation. I have a colleague who is naturally lean and who finds it very difficult to be sympathetic toward our very overweight patients. When she put a handmade sign up in our waiting room that said FAT KILLS! I knew there was going to be trouble. Our entire office staff found it way too harsh and made her take it down. As the most confident and outspoken full-figured gal in the group, and as someone who has a great relationship with this practitioner and shares her sense of humor, I approached it differently from almost everyone else. I told her I thought it was an inappropriate way to manage her jealousy over my figure. Fortunately, because of our mutual respect and similar sense of humor, this launched us into a serious conversation about weight and how to be most helpful to patients whose appetites had gone haywire. Of note: this constructive conversation took place over lunch, which for her consisted of Pringles and a bottle of Mountain Dew. She, like many physicians, works very long hours, doesn't get enough sleep, eats junkfood, has limited knowledge of nutrition, and only gained weight when she was pregnant—and then lost it afterward. And, like everyone, she enjoys foods that aren't necessarily healthy and low calorie; she just happens to be someone who doesn't gain weight when she eats them. I understand how she feels about our population of patients who weigh in at well over 300 pounds. She just isn't the best person to talk with them about weight loss. A medical doctor may not be your best bet for good advice. Perhaps an exercise physiologist or an experienced integrative nutritionist (rather than a dietitian) would be a better choice. Whoever you choose, make sure he or she enjoys the work, is patient, and has a good and kind sense of humor. Pointing folks in a different and more self-empowered direction takes finesse and a real interest in the subject. It also absolutely demands paying close attention to their capabilities, lifestyles, and readiness for change. Taking a cookie-cutter approach to advising patients is highly depersonalized and rarely successful. Remember, the folks you hire for health care are on your payroll. If they're not meeting your needs and you don't feel like they understand what you're saying, then move on to someone else.

RETHINKING YOUR DEFINITIONS OF ATTRACTIVE AND SEXY

The many women tormented by their full figures who come to see me for sexuality counseling need to speak with my handsome, physically fit, and sexually sophisticated friend Eric. He's the man who told me that full-figured women are attractive in ways that lean women never will be *because* they're full figured and *not lean*. When Eric said this to me, it was like finally understanding quantum theory. This conversation was like my very own French Revolution, and very helpful personally and professionally. Imagine, the very flesh you loathe can be fetching, hot, and sexy! It also may be comforting to a partner who loves all of you, including those extra pounds you'd prefer to live without.

The IQ of foods and the joy of moving are the first things you need to reconsider. The next is your definition of beauty. Ask yourself who you consider attractive and appealing, and make a list of the reasons why you feel this way. If the only folks you can conjure up are your thin friends or movie stars, then go out into the world and do some people watching. Or look at some of the great lingerie catalogs for full-figured women. Look at everyone who goes by and find the features you like. Pay close attention to body types. Undoubtedly, you'll see folks who have bodies that you wouldn't want for yourself. That's fine. However, I guarantee you'll see people who don't fit your notion of the ideal or perfect figure but have other things that you find lovely and wish you had yourself. And by the way, they may very well be holding hands with their special someone.

Women need to think of themselves as whole packages. Our souls, personalities, and complex identities are woven into our physical beings. The wholeness is what others are attracted to and choose to stay near. If there were ever a living example of the concept that the whole is greater than the sum of its parts, it's the synergy that dictates the laws of attraction. Who you are in your entirety—bones, flesh, brain, and soul—and the stability and functionality of your markers of emotional well-being add or detract from your overall appeal, and this includes your sexiness.

Carving ourselves into separate pieces and critiquing each one—having too fat a belly, a smart-enough brain, ugly legs, a nice voice—undermines who we are as complex and unique individuals in our entireties. We don't function in the world as separate, disembodied parts, and no one sees or experiences us like that either, so what's the point of thinking of ourselves this way? Excessive focus on distinctly separate aspects of our selves "dis-integrates" us, deflects attention away from us instead of drawing it toward us, and can leave us dangerously preoccupied with ourselves. In an endless effort for self-improvement, we can wind up dismantling our capacity to function and experience pleasure in life through our senses by disengaging them from the whole of who we are. Doing this reduces us to self-criticizing shrews devoid of compassion for ourselves and attached to some false sense of perfection that is, at its core, not part of the human condition. In the name of self-improvement, we run the serious risk of forfeiting our full, in-color selves—warts included—for just one part of who we are. This way of thinking will not facilitate or enhance our relationships with pleasure, and there is nothing powerful about it either. In order to fully access both, you must bring your whole self to the table to feast, with unabashed intention, on as many of life's pleasures as possible—including food. Under optimal circumstances, you will do so simply because your humanness makes it possible to enjoy what life has to offer you—with no strings attached.

QUESTIONS TO ASK YOURSELF

1. What physical features do I have that I find attractive and appealing? What have others commented on as being attractive?

2. Why does my partner tell me he or she wants to have sex with me? Do I like the reason, and do I believe it?

3. What do I consider to be the attributes of the ideal woman's body—figure and face—and why?

4. Who do I know who doesn't fit the stereotype of the sexy woman, yet I and others find her attractive and alluring. Why?

5. Which of my physical features can I change (without surgery) and which are immutable?

6. How much of a role do I feel that physical and mental health play in whether or not I see myself as attractive?

7. What stops me from moving in the ways I want to and that I know would be better for my health? How can I change this?

CHAPTER 4

I JUST CAN'T RIGHT *NOW*

Everybody's heart is open, you know, when they have recently escaped from severe pain, or are recovering the blessing of health.

—JANE AUSTEN

America is known the world over as a powerful democracy and a land where just about anyone can achieve their dreams for a free and comfortable life. This has resulted in a long history of immigration of people representing a highly diverse array of cultures and mores from all over the world. But, despite the melting-pot demographics of the United States, the Puritan pilgrims and their philosophy of austerity had an indelible influence on the expressiveness of Americans. Generally, Americans are not known as people who openly weep and wail at funerals; jump out of cabs to yell directly in the faces of offending motorists; or employ culturally sanctioned, lengthy rituals and practices as coping strategies during difficult times. This emphasis on work is both good and bad—good for our gross national product, but bad for our mental health, and *really* bad for our sensual and sexual lives.

The fully inculcated American typically finds emotions much too complicated and untidy to give them all the room and time they really need to air out and dry. If you're a first- or second-generation immigrant from a culture that does wail at funerals and sanctions spending three hours over lunch every Sunday at the grand pooh-bah grand-mother's house, or if you need to take different days off for fasting, praying, and feasting than everyone else in your office, then you know what I mean. As a very ethnic Greek American, I am very familiar with this. I have always been something of a curiosity in the workplace for my different Easter schedule and my effusive and emotive personality. So much so that at one time, I was politely asked not to at-tend staff meetings because my communication style was just too much for my colleagues. Fortunately, my boss at the time was Greek American also, and when she delivered the news, she tempered it with "Don't worry about it. It's just the Greek thing." I calmed down immediately because I knew exactly what she meant: I was just too loud and too forceful, and I expressed my opinions with too much con-viction, and, more than anything else, *too much emotion.*

Like my Italian and Latin brethren, when I have some-thing important or meaningful to say, I use every part of my body to get my point across. I don't see the value of speaking in a normal tone of voice devoid of expletives and without gesticulation for emphasis. And, when I express joy or sorrow, my affect matches my sentiment. As an American citizen, I have had to learn to temper this. But it's not easy for me to pull back on my own reins. Even after nearly 20 years of marriage, my partner will sometimes look at me and ask me why I am acting upset and yelling when there's nothing really upsetting going on. My response: "I am *not* *yelling* or upset! What are you *talking* about?!" She then points out that Poseidon, were he 20,000 leagues under the sea, could hear me. Who knew? In my experienced opinion, I believe my method of coping with emotions indicates that I have exemplary mental health. I feel it, say it, and act it out with my body, and discharge the feelings, and then they're less likely to continue to upset me—or at least not as much. Real Americans? They use a different model.

The American way of managing feelings often involves round after round of psychotherapy with a stranger who may very well be just as troubled as the client seeking their services. However, the way the system is structured, there's no real way of knowing this ahead of time. Jonathan Alpert, a practicing psychotherapist in New York and the author of *Be Fearless: Change Your Life in 28 Days,* wrote a terrific opinion piece for *The New York Times* citing multiple studies that revealed the ineffectiveness of long-term therapy. In most cases, people improved after very few sessions and the rate of improvement actually decreased as the number of sessions increased. Nonetheless, some practitioners and patients alike will persist with their weekly or biweekly visits for years.[4] Seeing an experienced and well-trained psychotherapist for help with a psychological or emotional problem isn't inherently a bad idea. In cases where someone is struggling from a complicated and/or chronic psychiatric problem, medications and ongoing psychoeducational and supportive counseling can make the difference between coping well or not coping at all. But honestly and calmly talking with the people involved is an important first step. You might be surprised by how infrequently this actually occurs, especially between intimate partners.

A major reason folks come to see me as a sexuality counselor is because they are struggling with having sex or experiencing pleasure of any kind with the person they most want to have these experiences with. The number one question I ask them is whether or not they've told their partners what they've just told me. The usual answer to this is no. This is anathema to how I live and defies what I consider to be logic and common sense. At the risk of oversimplifying any individual's complex psychology, if I am struggling, everyone who knows me the world over knows something about it. My theory is that if we speak up to the *right* people and those people allow their affects to accurately reflect their feelings, we'll all be better off. If you're struggling with something upsetting, be upset, even if this takes longer than 50 minutes weekly to express.

When my own grand pooh-bah grandmother died at the age of 88, her best friend, a fellow octogenarian immigrant from the Greek island of Samos, draped herself over the open casket, sobbing loudly in front of the entire congregation. The patient mourners in line behind her took this in stride—they were all Greek too and knew their turns would come up soon enough. All I could think was *how completely appropriate.* This is Greek-style mourning. You would never see such a thing at a Lutheran service. My friend Jean Naggar, author of *Sipping from the Nile: My Exodus from Egypt,* credits this kind of behavior to "Middle-Eastern sensibilities." Jean grew up in Egypt and knew plenty of Greeks. When I listened to her book on a CD in my car,

I would find reasons to run long errands simply so I could absorb her understanding of what it's like to live in the land of feelings and nonstop sensuousness. Listening to Jean reinforced my self-righteousness about the way I act. Make no mistake about it, the ethnic groups that fearlessly feel and express their emotions—good and bad—often have coping mechanisms and rituals that make managing difficult times and gigantic life transitions easier. We also aren't hesitant to take people along with us for help and support. After all, who doesn't need a hand when the going gets rough?

In my sex counseling practice, I make it clear to people from the beginning that while I have plenty of experience and lots of good ideas, they have to be honest about what they feel if they want to find their way out of whatever conundrum and pain they're in. I also tell them that feeling sad, upset, troubled, and even miserable or numb are all part of life and the human condition; they are not necessarily reflective of psychopathology. Sometimes, simply staying put in these feelings for a while is the very thing they need to do in order to mend and resume living powerful, pleasurable lives. There are certain things we just can't rush, and the bigger the upset or changes we're facing, the longer this process might take.

The sweeping changes brought about by new motherhood, illness, and grief are not sexy states of mind. They are also examples of times when we need help catching our breath and regaining our sea legs with plenty of support from others who love us. Such leviathan life events can trigger acute losses of self-confidence, physical stamina and stability, and, perhaps most devastatingly, our senses of optimism and faith. As a midwife, mother, and sexuality counselor, I have seen this and know it to be true personally and professionally. The seismic shifts that rumble beneath our feet when new life is ushered in, when we face our own mortality, or when we grieve the loss of someone we loved are hard to avoid, outsmart, fully understand, and predict. This is not a time when our pleasure quotients are high or our sexuality is easily accessed. Our culture is so focused on getting jobs done, tending to tasks, and avoiding the untidiness of emotions—especially complex or sad ones—that we simply don't have a mechanism or much patience for managing the rough seas that can last for indefinite periods of time. Think about it: most employers grant six weeks of paid maternity leave, very limited sick time, and three days of bereavement leave. This amounts to almost no time, really, to cope with some of the most significant and meaningful events any of us will ever experience. I rarely see people's sexuality peeking through the dense fog of sweeping change and upset that characteristically accompany these times of beginnings and endings.

NEW MOTHERHOOD

So let's jump right in with a discussion of new motherhood. The national standard for sending new mothers home from the hospital is 24 to 48 hours after a vaginal birth or 72 hours following a cesarean delivery. This wasn't the case when I first became a maternity nurse and then a midwife. Way back then, the time to discharge was determined by the practitioner on call, giving experienced maternal-child–health specialists ample leeway to decide if mother and baby were well enough to leave the hospital and whether they had the knowledge, emotional stability, and resources to manage once they were home. When I would see women 24 hours after delivery, I always asked them questions about how they were feeling emotionally, whether or not they had support at home, how feedings were going, and if they felt able to manage at home with their new babies. If there was any doubt in my mind about what awaited them there or about how the mother herself was faring and what her skill set was, I took advantage of her inpatient status, deferred her discharge, and worked with my nursing colleagues to find ways to shore up her strengths and have her leave with as many tools as possible to manage with. If it seemed as though continued assessment and support would be helpful once she was home, I would write orders for a maternal-child visiting nurse to see her for the first two weeks postpartum. Those days are long gone. The insurance industry changed its coverage policy and mandated that maternity patients be discharged after 48 hours following an "uncomplicated" vaginal delivery—no matter how long or taxing that delivery may have been—and 72 hours after an uncomplicated cesarean birth. This policy is based in part on staffing issues in hospitals as well as on the need to reduce hospital costs for inpatient postpartum care, which hospitals often have to absorb, particularly in the case of uninsured or underinsured patients. Meanwhile, the availability of maternal-child visiting nurses and of insurance coverage for their services has been reduced dramatically over the past 15 years in most areas of the United States, as have funds for special programs for parents at risk. Now, when I write orders for discharge, it's really just a formality. Barring a medical complication, lengths of stay are dictated by insurance companies versus obstetric providers. All I can do is hope that family, friends, or neighbors can step in where a skilled nurse might have in years past. This is extremely frustrating for me and a cruel and sometimes dangerous situation for mothers, infants, and new families.

After I delivered my own daughter, I left the hospital 48 hours later, despite having a high fever from a viral syndrome that preceded her birth and a postpartum hemorrhage that left me exhausted and feeble. About a month later, I wasn't able to sleep when my daughter did, my tearfulness was interfering with my daily life, and I felt a distinct sense of joylessness about virtually everything except my baby. This was not just the baby blues that normally come and go within the first couple of weeks following delivery. I had a full-blown postpartum depression that became increasingly crippling as weeks passed. Finally, at ten months postpartum, when symptoms of anxiety had coupled with my depression and my sleep debt had reached an all-time high, I managed to find my way into the office of a perinatal psychiatrist, who took one look at me and couldn't help but see that I was falling to pieces. My skilled and compassionate psychiatrist convinced me to take medication and reassured me that it would be all right for my daughter to continue nursing, and that she would, in fact, fare best once I started feeling better myself. Based on the statistics we have, approximately 10 percent of new mothers experience a postpartum depression and those who have had any depression prior to pregnancy are at even greater risk. Until I started feeling better and my sadness and anxiety abated with supportive counseling and medication, searching for joy and pleasure or being sexual never crossed my mind. I hadn't felt filled with faith or optimistic in months. And I had no ability to deal with the normal ups and downs of life with a new baby. For those first ten months after delivery, there were days when all I could do was nurse my baby and get myself dressed.

You don't have to have postpartum depression to lose your ability to access pleasure. Frankly, just having a baby can do this to a woman, even the most competent among us. Strange as it may seem, the most amazing experience of our lives isn't necessarily the easiest or happiest one. Imagine this scene: There you are, feeling half-dead from either having pushed what felt like planet Earth through your vagina or having had major abdominal surgery. Lying next to you is your eight-pound baby, who is screaming its head off and demanding your attention. You can't sit easily because your hemorrhoids and overstretched perineum are throbbing, everything else aches, the thought of moving your bowels strikes terror in your heart, and your little bundle of joy grabs hold of your nipple like a variant of the South American piranha. Being a new mother can be so disorienting and upsetting sometimes that feeling sustained optimism, faith, resilience, or self-confidence is impossible, at least for the first few months. Further, it's unprecedented and enraging when you realize that a little baby whom you deeply love has taken over your world, reduced you to tears, and made you feel like an idiot. After all, by the time many of us have our children, we've grown accustomed to being very competent and proficiently managing entire offices, operating rooms, and even big companies. So how is it that a person who can't talk, read, or drive; wears a diaper; and needs to be carried everywhere, can reduce us to a puddle of tears? That's a baby for you. Babies are powerful beings and will stop at nothing to get their points across— especially when they're unhappy. This can unravel a woman's composure and confidence quicker than anything I have ever seen. Add to this the many well-meaning but misguided relatives and friends who don't hesitate to offer unsolicited advice about how you should do something and it's enough to make a woman put her baby in a basket, send it down the Nile, and then drink fast-acting poison. With this confidence crisis taking root, you can imagine how new motherhood and pleasure—especially sexuality—make for a combination like a fish on a bicycle.

Despite the obvious correlation between our sexuality and conception, the immeasurably intense and challenging experience of having children, especially your first, doesn't blend easily or well with seeing yourself as a sexually desirable and active woman. The mere mention of having sex is likely to incite a scornful, even violent reaction in an otherwise loving and gentle woman.

The normalcy of a woman's disinterest in sex after delivery has to be viewed with perspective. After all, what's a few months' hiatus from sex when your intention is to spend a lifetime together? It's at this time that the art of self-pleasuring and masturbation can and should be honed by a hungry partner. Non-child-bearing men and women need to simply accept that a sexual Sahara is the norm, and as a woman going through this, it is your job to let your partner know that this is the time to be taking care of his or her own needs, either in your loving company, with no expectation of you rising to the occasion or, if you prefer, in the shower all on his or her own. I don't blame desirous, eager sweethearts for their wholehearted efforts to cozy up to their partners in hopes that it will pay off. I'm just here to tell you that it's okay for you to let those hopes fall flat—just make sure to reassure your partner that this isn't something personal. Not wanting sex is simply one of the many phases you will have to endure, but it too will pass, just like your child cutting teeth or throwing tantrums will. And if it doesn't, explore your parenting styles and priorities together and make a point of taking time away from your baby. By six months, in the absence of a treatment-resistant postpartum depression or a baby that isn't well, it's a good and healthy plan to begin carving out time for yourselves as a couple and leaving your infant for several hours or even overnight with a responsible babysitter and plenty of breast milk in the freezer.

Below are three stories from women in my practice that illustrate the issues of new motherhood and its impact on sexuality. As you read them, imagine yourself in what they say and see whether or not you can relate to their experiences.

> The difference between how I felt during and after this pregnancy and my first is radical! I was 26 when I had my son. Now, at 34, I am so tired I can't believe it. For whatever reason, I wasn't getting pregnant after I had my first son, and we just ended up accepting this and decided that having one child was fine with us. We just assumed I wouldn't get pregnant again. When I did we were thrilled, but I never thought the experience would be so different. The sleeplessness is killing me! I am so tired and I don't have just one child now, I have two and their needs are very different. I can't just sit on the sofa and stare at my baby. I have to do things for my older child and our family too. I am exhausted. My husband is helpful but doesn't really understand why I am so spent. He also can't figure out why I don't want to have sex right now. He takes it personally, and that's not how I am intending it. Right now, I feel like I am still landing from the experience of giving birth and being a new mother to both my baby and our son. Sex is just not an option right now. —*Michelle, 36 (three months postpartum)*

I just didn't expect that having my children so close together would take this much out of me. I somehow thought it would be easier to do it this way, but it absolutely isn't. Two are still in diapers, and all of them are less than two years apart. I haven't had a full night's sleep in more than five years. I have either been nursing or pregnant and working through all of this, too. I am so exhausted all the time. Despite the fact that my husband is a great father and very helpful, there are times that the kids want me and only me. This is certainly true with the youngest, who is still nursing. There is no question that having sex right now just feels like one more thing to do and one more person hanging on me. I have tried explaining this to my husband, but he can't seem to see the correlation. He tells me that he's not the kids and that it's different. But it doesn't feel different to me. By the time I get into bed at night, I don't want anyone near my body. Not him or them. —*Angela, 40 (four months postpartum)*

I waited to have kids until after I had finished my education and gotten the job I had worked toward. I thought this was the best way to do things and that my financial security would make things easier. Now, nothing feels easy. My kids are four and one, and I am just beginning to be able to leave them for periods of time, and it's mostly because I am desperate to have time to myself. My relationship with my husband has really suffered from having kids, which is a sad commentary on raising a family, but it's the truth. We finally went away together recently and it was great. We slept in, had sex in the late morning, and just walked around for the afternoon before we headed home that following evening. I was really rejuvenated and felt more like myself than I had in years. We have to do this regularly, but once I got home I felt like the kids' needs were right back in my face. I can't imagine what I would do if they were closer in age. I wouldn't be able to manage. —*Charlotte, 36 (one year postpartum)*

Charlotte's experience is noteworthy. She had been working with me for a few weeks before I was able to convince her that the 4 or 6 x 36 plan was worth trying. When I saw her after she and her husband came back, she was rejuvenated and vowed to go away again every four to six weeks. Her youngest was still nursing and didn't lose his stride while she was gone. This is true with many nursing babies, whose dependence on breast milk at one year of age is not nutritionally based, but comfort based. The happy nursing baby is likely to go right back to the breast when you return, so leaving for 36 hours in an effort to regain your self and your sexuality shouldn't be viewed as off-limits.

Mothering babies and very young children is taxing, to be sure, and not all babies are created equal. The first six months are a critical time for mothers and infants to establish their emotional bonds and nursing success and to become accustomed to one another's presence and subtle communication systems. But beware of time passing. In terms of your baby's temperament, both the unsettled malcontent and the sanguine contemplative are more resilient than we may think. And both do best when their primary care providers are well in body and mind. This means meeting your own needs while also meeting theirs. But in this I'm talking about true needs. It's hard to interpret this when thinking of your own children, but frankly, the tendency of children in general is that if you give them one hour, they'll push for two. Give them two and they'll beg for four. This is the way they are.

What we often interpret as a need is not a need, but a desire. As babies age it's reasonable to expect them to have increasing tolerance for frustration over waiting for or doing without things they want but don't need. While there are opposing schools of thought on this and a new trend in the United States to adopt what's called attachment parenting,[5] which has mothers and babies together at all times for the first couple of years, as an experienced mother and midwife I don't believe this is necessary for healthy growth and development. Also, living this way can wreak havoc on parents' relationships. Having time for and access to pleasurable adult activities drops way off if you're in babyland all the time. Babies are loveable and engaging beings. They're also exhausting, and caring for them has a tedious and frankly unpleasant side to it. Finding anything pleasant in your day can be difficult if you're constantly doing things for your infant. Sometimes the best thing for both babies and mothers is for mothers to hand them over to someone else who can appreciate them because they're not with them every minute. This gives mothers an opportunity to refuel and come back to their infants when they're not as exhausted. This is especially true if your baby is difficult to soothe or problematic for whatever reason.

ILLNESS

Throughout my career in midwifery and sexuality counseling, I have encountered women of all ages who have marshaled their strengths and fought against debilitating illnesses and disabilities that demand all their attention and distract them from all that is good in life. These experiences leave me dazzled by women's courage to endure painful therapies and cope with the seemingly intolerable, all in the interest of resuming life as they once lived it, free of unrelenting fear of pain and premature death. It is humbling to bear witness to their stories and a great reminder that none of us should take our pleasures and capabilities for granted.

It's easy to see how pleasure and sex can disappear from a woman's life when she's facing the potential of a shortened life while also undergoing painful treatments, not to mention the responsibility she may feel to appear calm and in charge during this frightening and uncertain time. Many women who are facing illness put all of their energy and concentration into keeping their chins up for their own sakes as well as those of family members, including partners who are equally terrified by an uncertain outcome. This is a time when body betrayal and the fear it generates are the most dominant sentiments, with the woman asking herself over and over again, *how and why did this happen?* and *what's going to happen next?*

Despite the hair-raising terror and uncertainty of these times, plenty of women have an unflagging determination to manage and live as if nothing unusual were occurring. We all know at least one woman who, during a course of chemotherapy or very shortly after a major surgery, was sitting at her desk at the office as if nothing in her life had changed. That's the American spirit in action. Personally, barring a life-changing event that I can't miss, I go to bed when I am sick or exhausted. I also complain, whine, and sometimes even cry and ask that at least some of my needs be attended to. The idea that we should buck up and act as though we're sailing through calm seas when in fact we've hit a tsunami is bizarre and taxing. Some advocates of this approach claim that it's the best way to cope. If you don't let any fear or negativity infiltrate your thinking, you'll fare better. But there are casualties in this. While you're working every second to avoid thinking negative thoughts and feeling your fears, you're expending so much energy doing so that there's no opportunity for more pleasurable things to be fully experienced. Also, your determination to stay cheerful and upbeat may actually be dismantling your faith and optimism. I have seen people so wedded to a positive outlook that they lived with crippling denial about what was actually happening to them. The Pollyanna style might work for some, but it demands great effort to blunt normal emotions. When sick people pretend that everything is fine, it doesn't allow their upset to come to the surface, be expressed, and then dissipate, the way emotions are likely to do if they're expressed. The tide comes in and then it goes out again, and in between we enjoy the sea the way it is in the moment.

Most of the time, women come to me when their illnesses are in remission or have been cured and they're longing to regain some semblance of their former sexual selves. They tell me they simply don't know where to begin and feel like they've lost their sense of sexuality altogether. New normals, such as chronic pain syndromes, disfigurement, and an altered body image, or the need for altered living habits to accommodate medications or physical limitations, make it difficult to reimagine oneself as a sexually active person. Further, medical practitioners focused on curing easily lose track of the impact of diagnosis and treatment on their patient's sense of power in the world and of their sexuality. Sadly, interacting with practitioners and undergoing their curative therapies are often deeply depersonalizing experiences, leaving patients' psyches to fend for themselves. One of my patients related that when she tried to discuss difficulties she was having with intercourse as a result of her chemotherapy, her oncologist remarked, "What else do you want? You're alive. Isn't that enough?" This is a perfect example of how preserving someone's quality of life to the greatest extent possible while also curing the disease isn't always as important to practitioners as it is to patients.

While sex isn't necessarily in the foreground of people's minds if they're ill, the need for affectionate and loving touch often is, and it can prove to be the perfect on-ramp for bringing pleasure back into your life. And it can certainly help you rekindle your desire for sex and get your sexual mojo back. Skin-to-skin contact is soothing, curative, pain-relieving, and comforting. Being stroked and held by someone who loves you and whom you love in turn is therapeutic. The language of the hands can be deeply, lovingly expressive, and this touch often does more good than any conversation ever could. The impact on brain chemistry is divine, with the higher level of oxytocin resulting in muscle relaxation and an improved sense of well-being. A word of caution: if your intimate partner has also provided your nursing care, don't expect that resuming your sexual relationship will come easily. In fact, based on what I have seen in my practice, I highly recommend that your lover not be your nurse. Keep the boundary between intimate partner and personal care provider intact. Once you cross it, it's difficult to go back.

Below is a story from one of my clients who recovered from breast cancer and came to me after her treatment, including a mastectomy, was complete. Her prognosis was good, and her desire to regain her sexual self had surfaced.

Now that I have finished my chemotherapy and my hair and energy are beginning to come back, I'm feeling more like my old self, and I want to be sexual again. I feel like this is a new me in a way, and I feel like this is part of celebrating my health and the fact that I am alive and well. I'm still struggling with some of the lasting effects of surgery, and I worry sometimes that my husband is more upset about my breast not being there than he admits. But, he tells me over and over again that this isn't the way he feels, so I need to accept that he's telling me the truth; at least I hope he is. Anyway, things are what they are. When I was experiencing treatment, I was so focused on getting well that the thought of being sexual was so far away from anything on my mind. But now I don't feel this way, because I am relieved and hopeful about the future. I don't feel like my death is imminent or as likely in the near future as I did when I was first diagnosed, so doing the things I used to enjoy and that gave me pleasure—like having sex—feels possible again.
—Rita, 60

Chronic illnesses, versus acute ones, pose a complicated challenge for women because they are generally remitting-relapsing conditions that can flare up at any time and that almost always impair day-to-day function. Because these conditions never fully resolve and those who live with them often need to adopt habits that will minimize or still their symptoms, invariably, the condition impacts their sense of confidence as well as their general faith and optimism. Living while waiting for the other shoe to drop is stressful and can impose significant limitations. This is especially difficult with chronic pain syndromes like arthritis and fibromyalgia and bowel disorders like Crohn's disease, severe irritable bowel syndrome, and colitis. It is also true for mood or anxiety disorders. Chronic mental health problems can be especially difficult to live with because of the stigma attached to them and their impact on loving partners. Living with chronic depression alienates people and can seriously impact a loving relationship. Depression and anxiety frustrate those who are afflicted as well as those who love them, especially if many of the elements of a good life are present. The perceived illogic of depression in someone who has the ingredients for good and comfortable living can exacerbate both the symptoms and a mate's intolerance.

When I am working with a patient who has a condition that isn't curable but can be well managed, I need to know what relationship they've developed with their diagnosis in order to understand how their pleasure-seeking practices and sexual identity will fit into their life. When someone uses a medical diagnosis as their primary identifying feature, then pleasure will be harder to come by than if their diagnosis is in the background of their identity. My objective is to help women identify what works best to ameliorate their symptoms and to use these interventions to both plan for and encourage pleasure and sex. I recommend that women be honest with their partners about their constellation of symptoms while also maintaining their independence as patients in the management of their symptoms. Being treated like *the patient* will surely have a saltpeter effect on sexuality and pull you away from pleasure quickly and efficiently. Explain this to your partner and make sure he or she understands the difference between being helpful and smothering or infantilizing. Consider the following stories from two clients of mine. They have very different chronic conditions and yet their needs are very much the same when it comes to their sexual lives.

I can take care of myself and my symptoms. I have been doing this since I was a teenager, when I was first diagnosed. It makes me so angry and not at all interested in being sexual when my husband tries to be my nurse. I don't need that kind of help from him and if I do, I need to be the one to ask for it. When he treats me like a patient or as if I am so delicate that he can't get near me, it accentuates the fact of my illness and the symptoms and leaves me feeling much more aware of them than when I am left to manage them on my own. I am a grown woman, can take care of myself, want to take care of myself, and don't need to be treated like an invalid. And anyway, invalids don't have sex. I want to have sex and my disease doesn't need to be the center of attention all the time. —Aisha, 37

I have struggled with depression my whole life. It started when I was a teenager, and eventually I was diagnosed with bipolar depression. My moods can fluctuate rapidly. Fortunately, I have been stable on my medications for about nine years and my mood shifts aren't as frequent or as intense as they used to be. But the way my partner manages with these fluctuations can leave me feeling anything but interested in having sex. There are times when I may feel something intensely—like passion for example—and this will make her suspicious—as if all my intense feelings are to be attributed to being bipolar. Whether I have a mood disorder or not, I still have the capacity to feel things deeply, just like other people who don't have bipolar depression. I know I can't separate myself from my diagnosis but my personality isn't solely based on my psychiatric diagnosis. I don't always want to be seen as the partner with a "condition." And anyway, I manage my condition well on my own. There isn't anyone who knows more about my wide range of feelings than I do. I just want to be taken for who I am in my entirety and not parceled into my mood and my other self. This includes whether I am interested in sex or not. —*Elizabeth, 52*

Any chronic illness demands ongoing tending to by the person afflicted as well as their loved ones. There are ways to do this effectively, including maintaining a focus on appreciation for when things are going well and a sincere willingness to immediately address any symptoms of a relapse before it grows in size and force. This usually depends on how intelligent, insightful, and honest someone is with themselves and others and the extent to which they have been educated by their health care provider about how best to manage their condition. Relapses are difficult to face. Their unknown endings are frightening to people and discourage them, especially when things have been going well and the most distressing manifestations has been quiet for long periods of time. The wavelike pattern of the symptoms of chronic conditions is unavoidable. The grace with which we manage them is the defining factor as to how intrusive they become and whether we define ourselves by our ailments or not.

GRIEF

I have experienced death as both a deafening, unexpected explosion that threw me off my feet as well as something I opened the door for and welcomed in like an old friend. Whether unexpected or welcomed, in both cases I found myself preoccupied for varying periods of time with these questions, *where has my loved one gone, what will life be like without them,* and *how do I grieve this loss?*

Regardless of your religious upbringing or current beliefs about an afterlife, human beings look to ritual, ceremo-
ny, and one another to help manage with the knowledge
we will never again be able to see, speak to, or hear the
voice of a person we were attached to and loved. While
volumes of material have been written about death, dying,
and grief, processing and managing the death of someone
you loved remains one of the most uniquely personal experiences each of us will have.

And death is not the only loss that people respond to
with grief. Any big transition, including the loss of a job
(and the status it gives us), a relationship, good health, or
someone we love who's moved away, can trigger a grief
response. There is no right or wrong way to grieve. It var-
ies from person to person—the amount of time needed
and the coping mechanisms used are very individual. But
based on my experience in practice, those grieving do have
something in common—if grief is close to the surface, has
been ignored, or its magnitude has been understated, it
will unequivocally trump any desire for pleasure. Any unstoppable and irreversible change that affects life can also
trigger intense feelings of powerlessness.

The all-encompassing features of great loss, its incessant drone and persistent high-beam lights, can make us
deaf and blind to the gestures and voices around us, even
those of someone who deeply loves us and craves our re-
surfacing from the underworld of sadness and mourning.
When I have worked with couples whose sexuality has all
but vanished following the death of a woman's parent, for
example, I have seen over and over again how the expectation for sex can be devastatingly distancing. Sometimes
it's the overwhelming nature of grief, especially early on,
that keeps a woman away from the vibrant, life-filled act

of making love. Other times, a kind of survivor's guilt takes hold that won't allow a woman to say yes to pleasure, especially the sensual confluence of full-body, skin-to-skin contact that is exclusive to our living realm. I often think of this as the grieving woman's way of sharing the experience of death with the one she's lost, the one who no longer has access to human experience. Regardless of the reasons, pleasure is rarely thought of and sexuality is rarely expressed when someone is deeply grieving. Not acknowledging this is a dangerously negligent stance on the part of the less grief-stricken partner. Below are the words of a client who had lost her father, the parent she was closest to and whose absence she was finding very hard to recover from:

> My relationship with my father was always close. Because my mother was so unloving and so cold in general, to everyone really, his love for me and his warmth compensated for what she wasn't able to give, and the result through the years was that I looked to him—and he to me, I think—for a kind of support and attention that most people probably get from their marriages. It has been difficult for me to manage with his death and to feel recovered. I don't know if this is normal grief, but I feel like no one wants to hear about it anymore and that everyone has the expectation that I should be fine by now. I am not fine. I think I have been doing a lot of stuffing of my feelings because I am afraid of people's criticism, so I go through life pretending that I am fine when I'm not. This has been especially true with my husband, and it has definitely impacted our sexual life. I have absolutely no desire or interest in having sex, and at this point I wonder whether or not it's partially out of spite. I have felt like my husband, of all people, should be understanding about my grief but he isn't, so I have

felt myself shut down completely to him. It's created so much tension, but I am angry and I can't seem to shake this anger long enough to feel anything else, especially any sexual interest. —*Kate, 60*

The story below is from someone who came to see me after she sold a successful company that she started. She found herself retired at the age of 50.

I sold my company about a year ago. At first, the freedom was great! I was so thrilled when I realized that I had achieved my goal of retiring at 50. This is what I was working toward when I started the company in my late 20s. But now that the initial excitement has passed, I am lost and I don't have any idea of what to do with my life. I don't have anywhere to be every day, my time is completely unstructured, I feel like I have no purpose in life. I can't find a purpose in life. This is not at all what I expected. I miss the community of people I worked with and the sense of belonging it gave me. I feel like a young woman still. I don't know what I thought I would be like at 50 but playing golf every day and sitting around reading the newspaper is definitely not what I want to be doing right now. I am sad, and I never imagined I would feel this way. And the toll it's taking on my marriage is big. We've been fighting and the idea of being close or having sex is impossible for me to imagine. —*Julia, 50*

The best explanation I have ever heard about how people cope with grief came from my colleague Marcia Bernstein, an exceptionally talented mental health practitioner who has worked with grieving in her practice and studied grief professionally. In one of our conversations about the grieving process, she said, "You grieve, grieve, grieve—and then you go to lunch." If only grieving individuals and those who love them could take this in stride and let grief follow its own course, we would all be better off. In Kate's case, she felt rushed, silenced, and criticized for how her grieving process was shaped. As a consequence and as a way of honoring it, she made it her constant companion, leaving little room for anything or anyone else. This resulted in an enormous amount of dissatisfaction in her life and a huge distance between her and her husband that resulted in months of celibacy as a couple. In Julia's case, the fact that her success had ended up leaving her grief stricken only compounded the upset she felt and made creating a new life a burden, not something to celebrate. She felt the loss deeply and was embarrassed that this was the case. She didn't know what to do next and felt frozen in time, without any sense of what direction to move in.

Neither Kate nor Julia was able to move back from their grief into a more active and satisfying life. What they were experiencing was dark and leaden and included an element of embarrassment about how they felt. Going to their partners with this was not proving successful and felt burdensome to both women. It also seemed to be interfering with and delaying their recovery process. These situations occur more commonly than you might think, and what Kate and Julia experienced was not atypical of what goes on for many people when faced with a major life change.

The Recovery Process

There are occasions when the intense emotions from life's upheavals become so omnipresent that you might consider them abnormal. In these cases, seeking the assistance of a mental health provider who has experience working with grieving or depressed patients is a sound and helpful choice. This is a time when problem-focused short-term psychotherapy or the help of a support group is totally appropriate. I am not talking about seeing someone for months or years on end. But, affording yourself the time and space to talk about your sadness or feelings of powerlessness with an objective listener or others who can identify with your feelings can be very helpful. Sometimes, when you are convinced there is nothing that will alleviate your heartache or your stress, a completely objective and intelligent audience can offer a suggestion that never crossed your mind or that of anyone else you've shared your feelings with. It also takes the pressure off your intimate partner. When grief or postpartum depression that is expressed stridently hangs on, it's not easy for our partners to manage both our feelings and their sense of losing us to these same emotions. Having a safe and contained space where you allow your deepest sorrows and worries to be openly aired regularly and for structured amounts of time gives you a chance to express your feelings without being criticized or feeling like you're imposing on someone. This kind of help can assist you in organizing your emotional chaos into a more manageable package. Eventually, the loosely tethered bundle you've been lugging that keeps falling apart and tripping you can be placed in its rightful spot and you can move forward with less of a burden.

New motherhood, illness, and grief rob us of experiencing pleasure in our bodies. They make it difficult to connect with our capacity to feel joy by eclipsing it with their magnitude and breadth. They catapult us into an emergency-coping mode that demands we attend only to the most necessary things in order to simply stay upright, and by doing so, they can slowly erode our senses of empowerment and confidence. Self-empowerment's roots are in our capacity to soothe ourselves. Experiences that change our reality, identity, and sense of day-to-day life dramatically interrupt the rhythms we've developed to manage with all we knew before. Slowly, as you're forced to adapt to life's unpredictable and inevitable stressors, you can regain your ability to enjoy the pleasures that life offers, and this will be what helps you regain your sexual self. How long this takes and the precise course you'll take to get there will unfold as you live in and with your grief honestly. Some women incorporate massage into their routines on a weekly basis, reacquainting themselves with the pleasures of touch with no expectations attached. Others I've known have resumed playing an instrument or gone back to a dance class, where the music and movement usher them back to living in their bodies and enjoying them. Aromas and colors are another effective way to begin the process of retrieval—wearing different fragrances, repainting a room, or having a heady bouquet of roses on your night table regularly—no special occasion necessary—can awaken you (literally) after an understandable and sometimes seemingly interminable emotional slumber. And never forget the benefits of pets. The joyful company and therapeutic presence of animals in our lives can make the difference between feeling bereft 24/7 and having a sense of purpose and pleasure in life—at least some of the time. This may sound too elementary or simplistic. But we all have to begin with something as we slowly unfurl and reconnect with ourselves and others. As we add more and more sensual pleasures back into our daily lives, we're better able to regain our optimism, faith, confidence, and feelings of power in life. Pleasure—in its many forms—will begin to come back into the foreground while our challenges and grief slip slowly backward, assuming their rightful place. Whether we fully recover from losses or simply adapt to them really doesn't matter. I think the issue is more that we need to make room for them in our lives and live in some kind of harmony with change regardless of the size and force of the temblor.

QUESTIONS TO ASK YOURSELF:

1. Is there a challenge in my life that I have allowed to become my constant companion at the expense of my loving relationship? If so, why, and what can I do to change this?

2. How do I perceive myself as a mother, and what is its impact on my relationship with my partner?

3. Other than my partner, who else can I look to for help in managing life's difficulties?

4. What pleasures can I always count on to comfort me when sadness and/or grief feel dominant?

5. Am I aware of the impact that deeply upsetting events have on my sense of power and my ability to experience life's pleasures, including sexual intimacy?

6. Am I willing to ask for professional help when I face changes that I find very hard to manage? If not, why?

CHAPTER 5

MENOPAUSE IS KILLING ME

*There are some things you learn
best in calm, and some in storm.*

—WILLA CATHER

Many of the women I have worked with as a midwife and sexuality counselor have been women between the ages of 45 and 55. I have grown to refer to this decade in women's lives, including my own, as our personal Decade of Hell, a new ring of *Dante's Inferno* that we each discover and are immersed in for a full ten years until menopause and true middle age are behind us. When I meet for the first time with a woman who is somewhere along this continuum, I prepare myself for hearing reports of the following: tumultuous changes, big challenges, and extraordinary acts of courage. The gladiators don't hold a candle to women in this decade when it comes to charging into battle, taking on demons, and slaying dragons that happen to cross their paths. Without the protection of a battalion, armor, or a trusty lance, the midlife woman often faces her opponents head-on with nothing more for weaponry than her wisdom, pragmatism, and a sense of urgency to make the best of the second half of her life. For many of the women I see, a common enemy to leading a pleasurable life and feeling their power in it is a deep well of sexual dissatisfaction and lost sexual identity. In the course of raising children, building a career, and managing a household, it is not uncommon for the midlife woman to come to the realization that her sexuality has been on the back burner for years and that this has bothered her more than she's wanted to admit. And, for the women whose sexuality has remained vibrant and accessible despite the demands of work and family, normal midlife changes in biology and psychology that affect sexuality can feel disconcerting and worrisome. Either way, women between the ages of 45 and 55 are often thinking seriously about sex and its meaning and place in their lives.

The first half of my Decade of Hell went swimmingly and the changes and challenges I experienced were welcomed, promising, and long hoped for. Then, capsizing waves hit, and I too was facing what I had heard so many midlife women speak of: unexpected and troubling career issues, a marked loss of stamina, very uncomfortable perimenopausal symptoms, and losses I couldn't have predicted. I also noticed that for the first time in my life, my sexual vitality had decreased dramatically—and this started to affect all of my pleasure-seeking behaviors. I was facing exactly what so many of the women who come to see me had been describing: I was living in the land of *no*—no energy, no desire, no sex.

We can use the courage, fortitude, and creativity that midlife grants us to redefine what sexuality means and work with our changing bodies and psyches to continue living sexually satisfying lives. Or, we can throw in the towel and conclude that having great sex—or any sex, for that matter—is too much work and should remain a thing of the past. This is the choice we all face. Personally, I have loved sex for too long to let it go easily. My devotion to pleasurable and powerful living as a way to keep sex alive, interesting, and appealing has never faced a greater opponent than midlife. So, let's get started.

MENOPAUSE IS NOT A DISEASE, BUT IT CAN BE A MONSTER

There have been countless times in both my gynecology and sexuality counseling practices when women blamed menopause for everything that ailed them. This tendency to attribute nearly all illnesses, bad moods, and untoward outcomes to haywire hormonal activity reflects a ubiquitous misunderstanding of what's going on with our hormones in the first place. I often wonder how it is that so many women have such gross misunderstanding of even the basics of their own physiology. Even well-educated women are forever attributing all their midlife struggles to hormonal irregularity. To me this is a bit like sugar being responsible for hyperactivity in children. As an informed practitioner and perimenopausal woman, I am here to tell you that neither your hormones nor Twinkies will alter your judgment to such an extent that murder becomes a reasonable choice. Both may leave you feeling tired, irritable, bloated, and unappealing, but blaming everything that ails you on your ovaries (or a packaged snack cake) reveals serious flaws in your knowledge of body chemistry and how you can both manage and even capitalize on various unpleasant and challenging symptoms.

Menopause is defined by having gone 12 consecutive months without a menstrual period. The average age that this occurs at for American women is 52. Perimenopause marks the two to ten years preceding that point in time, and that is when most women feel the distress they refer to as *menopause*. Hot flashes, PMS, bloating, new food sensitivities, sleep disturbances, memory loss, fatigue, "fuzzy brain," changes in fat distribution, mood instability, decreased libido, and changes in vaginal lubrication and elasticity are common complaints of women whose ovaries are preparing for retirement or already collecting a pension. The medical term for this is *ovarian failure*. In my opinion, no one's ovaries actually fail. They simply kick back on a figurative chaise lounge and grab a martini; recount all the periods, pregnancies, and mental-health days they've given you; and decide it's time to quit working so hard. The eventual outcome is no menses at all, which marks the onset of menopause. After 12 months of no period, you are officially postmenopausal. Most women I know are relieved—if not thrilled—when their periods finally stop and mad as hell about the changes that come with it. Gals, you can't have it both ways!

There is no doubt that some women's perimenopausal and postmenopausal symptoms can be very hard to live with. If you're one of the unfortunate women who self-immolates on a regular basis, can no longer wear silk because of embarrassing perspiration stains, or is having malarial-level night sweats with consequential sleep interruption, then you know what I mean. Or, if you changed to an extra-large pocketbook to accommodate your feminine products because your monthly menstrual flow mimics the flooding Mississippi, then there's no question that this time of life is highly inconvenient, to say the least. Or, maybe you're like I am and that *special* time of the month makes you cry when the UPS man gives you a genuine hello because somehow you've come to believe that he's the only person who's been nice to you—ever. Or, if you bloat so much that your loving partner can't help but tell you the distortion makes you look a bit like Humpty Dumpty. And then there is the word-retrieval problem that's added to the rest of the memory loss, and by this time you're looking up "signs of Alzheimer's" on the Internet and scheduling an evaluation. As I said . . . it can be a monster.

If you're postmenopausal and like the majority of women, then you'd probably come to see me in my mid-wifery practice because penetrative sex feels like you're being impaled on a fence post, you're sporting snake skin, and you're hoping that modern medicine has come up with a gravity-defying pill as an alternative to a breast reduction and lift. These are embarrassing, distracting, and some-times limiting symptoms that press every panic button we have about aging. If you're struggling with these symptoms to the point of impaired living versus simple annoyance, then this is the time for better living though chemistry. Go to a well-informed and experienced health care provider and get medicine or hormones to help relieve your suffer-ing. Hormone therapy and maybe something you never thought of, such as nutritional supplements or a dietary ad-justment, can mean the difference between living a com-fortable life and not. You don't need to stay on the stuff for the rest of your life, and actually you probably shouldn't.

But hormone replacement therapy in various forms can make all the difference in the world and is a completely appropriate way to bridge perimenopause and menopause. In some cases, certain types of hormone therapy—like topical vaginal estrogen to maintain vaginal and urological health and comfort—are the best things we have to offer aging women. As for your nonpharmaceutical options, there are plenty, including staying physically active, eating well, having a good social network, getting adequate sleep, staying calm, and being willing to inform the people you live and work with that you're having a difficult time and would appreciate their TLC. And do your best to find the humor in it! (Let's just say that Humpty Dumpty comment may have actually been said to me.) However, I think the most important tip I can give is to remember that many of these symptoms will pass and, while you may be uncomfortable and inconvenienced, menopause is not a disease. No one goes into hospice care because they are perimenopausal. Your job is to decide what you need help with, find a skilled person to give it to you, and pay attention to your overall health for the rest of your life, which will take more effort and time than ever before.

The biggest culprit in perimenopausal symptoms is not necessarily the decreasing estrogen in and of itself, but the shift in the ratio and amounts of both estrogen and progesterone and the fact that this change doesn't follow a slow and even course of decline. The combination of a change in the ratio—with progesterone becoming more dominant at times—and a sometimes erratic pattern of hormone levels can create all sorts of uncomfortable symptoms that don't abate until menopause actually occurs. I don't feel dispassionate toward women's suffering, and I certainly do plenty of my own bellyaching when my perimenopausal symptoms clobber me and won't let up. However, if this is my biggest problem in life, oh well. It's much better than many of the other options out there—serious illness, homelessness, and nuclear war, for example. Your attitude is what will make the difference as to whether or not you experience this time of life as a death knell or an opportunity for expanded and pleasurable living in all areas of your life, including sex. Stay focused on the great things you do have, the absence of certain problems you've been able to solve, and, most of all, your best accomplishments and what they will allow you to do now. In my case, I had successfully put my daughter through college debt-free for both of us—all on my own—and she finished by the time she was 21 and I was 52. This meant that a huge financial pressure had been lifted from my shoulders and the demand to make as much money as when she was in school was gone. I was both really proud of this accomplishment—for me and for her—and thrilled that I could now work less because college costs were a thing of the past.

IN COMES PERIMENOPAUSE, OUT GOES MY FIGURE, MY BRAIN, AND MY SEXUALITY

One morning, I woke up, looked in the bathroom mirror, and said out loud, "What the fuck happened last night? I *know* I didn't go to sleep with *this* body. Who came and moved my fat around?!" For whatever reason, that particular morning I noticed on my own body the redistribution of fat that my midlife patients question and complain about all the time. I had lost about 50 pounds ten years before and was proud of the fact that I had successfully kept it off. Now, it appeared as if some of the fat was returning—but not exactly. I wasn't really any fatter, but my fat had definitely been newly distributed. My partner, who is five years older and more experienced, started to laugh and took great pleasure in reminding me of my age and what I have always known: fat distribution changes with age and, like it or not, we sport a fleshier belly and leaner upper chest wall, upper arms, and, sometimes, face and neck. And as for our breasts, well, they too lose fat and collagen, making them oh-so-deferent to Newton's law of gravity. While the fleshier belly part is very unappealing to most of us, it actually has an important function: it stores estrogen that protects our bones, vaginas, and brains as we get older. Fat is an endocrine gland. In other words, it stores and secretes hormones which can work for us or against us, depending on how much of it there is and where exactly it is located. Too little fat can contribute to problems like osteoporosis. Too much makes heart disease, diabetes, and some cancers more likely to develop. From the looks of it that morning, I was an estrogen swamp and sure to face a premature death from something related to having more fat than was optimal. Furthermore, while I was perfectly accepting of it on the bodies of my 50-and-over patients, I couldn't come to terms with it on my own body. Like so many midlife women, I couldn't help but repeatedly go to that dark and imposing place that threatens our sexual vitality: *I am unattractive because I am old, which means I am too old to have sex. No one who looks like this is sexually attractive, and anyway, I've lost interest in it so what difference does it make?* This was a very difficult morning for me.

The fact that our bodies are changing so much in midlife is made worse by the fact that we feel as though we're losing our minds, too. I can't count the number of times I have walked from one room in my house to the next with a specific mission in mind, only to arrive at my destination with no idea of what I wanted to do there. This is annoying and wastes a lot of my time. A colleague who is an excellent internist and midlife woman herself reminded me of how difficult it is to think clearly when your sleep is so often interrupted by night sweats and a mind full of decisions to make; oh, excellent point. With so many of us tossing and turning when we're supposed to be sleeping, throwing covers on and off, and doing e-mails at 3 A.M. instead of counting sheep, it's a wonder we can remember anything. Then, the depression sets in because the sleep debt has mounted, and you're tearful over everything and nothing. By this time, we're certain that mental clarity is a thing of the past and we're on the slippery slope toward dementia. All kidding aside, it's a rough ride when you can't come up with simple nouns like *shoulder, train, brisket,* and *poodle.* On the other hand, it's hilarious if you choose to let it be. What's most important to remember is that this symptom passes. Once women's sleep settles down because menopause has occurred, their word retrieval and low moods improve and they actually may end up being smarter than they were before.

In her book *The Secret Life of the Grown-Up Brain,* Barbara Strauch discusses the work of many researchers who are examining the particulars of brain function and health in midlife and beyond. When I saw this book, I grabbed it with a kind of desperation I knew was driven by my own worry about what might be going on upstairs that I needed to brace myself for. I was relieved to discover that many researchers she interviewed have found that our midlife brains do show evidence of wisdom and a greater ability to filter out negative concepts and choose positive ones instead. In the book Linda Fried, dean of Columbia

University's Mailman School of Public Health, says, "As you get older you can draw on objective knowledge and life experience and perhaps even intuition and they all get integrated and we can be more creative and solve complex problems that we could not solve when we were younger."[6]

Meanwhile, regardless of how much creative problem-solving prowess you supposedly have now that your brain is a half-century or more old, it doesn't seem to be making you any more interested in sex with your James or Jill Bond, which makes you wonder: *Will I ever want to have sex again?* This question might be haunting you, and even though you may wish your mind and perhaps your partner would shut up about it already, you can't help but wonder what the answer is. By now, you're probably thinking that this is all about your hormones. So, you make your way back to my office, certain that modern medicine must have *something* like Viagra for women. Or maybe you should just try Viagra—after all, it worked for Bob Dole and your best friend's husband. So what about testosterone?

TESTOSTERONE IS NOT THE HOLY GRAIL

Testosterone and its role in women's sexual desire has gotten quite a bit of press over the past several years. *The pink Viagra* is what folks in both the lay and medical communities started to call it. There was so much interest that, of course, big pharma started clinical trials to see if making such a thing in patch form might be the answer to turning women's switches back on. The excitement and backlash were equal, with the backlash winning out in the end. Despite the accelerated effort by Procter & Gamble, the Intrinsa patch died in phase III clinical trials and never did get off the ground. Nonetheless, supplemental testosterone has been prescribed off-label by many of us in the women's health-care field for years, but we've never had a specific United States, FDA-approved product designated for this purpose.

The science about how testosterone works to increase sexual desire in women isn't complete, but we do know that levels of testosterone decrease with menopause—just as those of estrogen and progesterone do. Without the physical and behavioral cues of reproductive biology leading women to want to have sex when they're fertile and making it more comfortable to do so, it's easy to see why midlife and postmenopausal women aren't that interested in sex—except when they have an affair or fall in love, which defies all we know about the role of reproductive biology in stimulating women's sexual desire—important food for thought.

As a practitioner and theorist on what makes women want sex at all, I have found that it's only a small percentage of my patients who really benefit from supplemental testosterone for improved desire. These are women who either don't have any ovaries due to having had a complete hysterectomy or have ovaries that have been damaged by chemotherapy or disease. Some women on selective serotonin reuptake inhibitor/(SSRI) antidepressants can benefit too, as these medicines suppress testosterone production. All total, this accounts for maybe 3 percent of my patients. Instead, the majority of women I see who complain of low libido are best served when they examine their lifelong relationships to pleasure and sex and also the status of their markers of emotional well-being as midlife women. If you're a midlife woman who can't see anything beautiful about who you are at your age and time of life, then you'll be a prisoner in celibacy jail forever. On the other hand, if you face the challenges of midlife with curiosity, humor, and a generous pinch of urgency to live life to the fullest, then midlife is replete with opportunities to sophisticate your sex life in ways that you simply didn't need to when you were younger and had more stamina, plenty of biological support, and a long life ahead of you. Fortunately, because so many midlife women are examining the quality of their lives anyway, throwing sex into the mix is relatively easy, and most women are game. And luckily, there's evidence that this reevaluation works.

I had a client once who came to me to talk about her sex life. She wanted to make things as exciting as possible and, frankly, things were pretty hot already. She was 75, sexy, and had a very big sexual appetite. In fact, she told me that after the first night she had had intercourse with her then-new partner, she was so thrilled about it that she did a little dance while walking her dog and said to herself, out loud, "I can't believe it, I got fucked last night!" This was a whoa-baby moment for me if there ever was one. I took this comment to heart and learned quite a bit from this patient about how fabulous sex can feel at any age regardless of how much testosterone you have circulating through your bloodstream. And she wasn't the only one. I have had many other women between the ages of 50 and 90 tell me that they thought sex was over for them until their children finally left the house, or untilthey met a new partner, retired from a job they hated, or were successful at a new endeavor they had taken on. These various shifts in life patterns and personal identities resulted in all sorts of changes, including having more sex than ever—and wanting it. None of these women had much circulating testosterone, but they were all living with healthy markers of emotional well-being, which made them able to access pleasure and find ways of making sex satisfying.

My theory is that when hormones decline, which all hormones naturally do with aging, conscious hedonism— a genuine willingness to try new things and a good sense of humor—should take their place and is more than capable of compensating for changes in biology. With so many legitimately upsetting limitations and losses facing us in midlife and beyond, we need to continually identify and harvest whatever pleasures we find, prioritize them as part of daily life, and include sex in the mix. Furthermore, it doesn't always have to be great sex or what I refer to as *life-threatening sex*. Plenty of times, maintenance sex will do. Just doing something that lets you know that all the parts still work and that you still enjoy your lover's touch and intimate company can be enough to leave you feeling better about your body and your partner. The fact that we're facing the last half of our lives in our late 40s and 50s— and there's no half after the last one—can make pleasure seeking easier to devote ourselves to. We no longer have to worry as much about the future; it's all about the present.

So when you start thinking about magic potions, you need to pause, take a step back, and reread the Introduction and Chapter 1 of this book. Review my premise that pleasure begets pleasure and determine which of your markers of emotional well-being are off-kilter. There is nothing quite as effective as the emotional and physical chaos of perimenopause and midlife to tip your scales away from accessing even easy, simple pleasures such as reading, taking a walk, or going to bed at a reasonable hour. When your midlife body feels like it's killing you and your brain seems to have stopped working altogether, don't take on anything complicated to start the ball rolling back in the direction of a pleasurable life. Call a massage therapist, take yourself out to your favorite healthy restaurant, or listen to music you love. And do it over and over again until you're back in the swing of things. When my body and brain feel their worst, that's when I force myself to go out for a walk, stretch, or swim. These remind me that all is not lost if I am still able to participate in things I really love and have the terrific side effect of helping me feel better. As you reestablish the balance of your emotional wellness, more pleasures will be easier to access, you'll feel more empowered, and sex may end up being right around the corner.

Management Strategies for Real-Life Changes

In order to have sex at all in midlife or beyond, you'll need to harness three critical concepts: 1) Pleasure has an inherent power that will make you feel your best. 2) Creativity is critical to being sexually satisfied at midlife and beyond. 3) Humor is your best lubricant for both 1 and 2. All three of these facts must be embossed on your thinking and active at all times in order to keep sex alive and breathing.

What you find pleasurable changes over time, and this is especially true as we age. Perhaps you've memorized the Kama Sutra, implemented all the positions, and always enjoyed Academy Award–winning thrusting. Now, your hip replacement, vaginal dryness, and staying power are sounding alarm bells at the mere thought of how things used to be. Or, maybe your antidepressant medication has impaired your ability to reach orgasm as easily as you used to. You feel like you're right on the edge, but just can't fall into that abyss of good vibes that you'd always been able to access before. Or, maybe your vaginal dryness and constriction keep steering you away from intercourse with your male partner altogether and you can't seem to come up with any alternatives. Now what?

Sexual fantasies, sex toys, and sexual aids enhance sexual experiences at any age and can be especially helpful when anatomy and physiology undermine or alter how we're accustomed to having sex. This is especially true for long-term couples when sexual ennui is killing both of you but you don't dare speak of it.

For many women, maintaining vaginal health is a major problem that starts at midlife, and it is grossly undertreated by practitioners in women's health. Despite the fact that vaginal changes are common, it is estimated that less than 25 percent of women who experience vaginal problems receive the treatment they need to relieve their discomfort and restore their genital health.[7] This is attributable to two factors: patients' discomfort in bringing their symptoms up and practitioners' discomfort in talking about sex. When the estrogen level drops, the vagina becomes less lubricated and much less elastic, making it painful for women to have penetrative sex. In addition, the introitus—the vaginal opening—narrows and the vagina itself shortens, which adds to women's discomfort. This can be even worse if you never had a vaginal birth or a hysterectomy, which would have allowed some helpful and lasting stretching of the vaginal tissues to occur. The use of vaginal estrogen products—suppositories, creams, or an indwelling ring that secretes small amounts of estrogen continuously—can make the difference between being able to enjoy your genitals or not. In addition, topical estrogen, as opposed to oral estrogen, has not been associated with an increased risk of breast cancer. In order to benefit from this treatment, you have to see a health care provider who is willing to work with you to find the treatment best suited to your needs. There is no one-size-fits-all solution for this, and it can take time to find the most effective regimen. But the clock is ticking, because the less penetrative sex you have, the more problematic it is to have it at all. Be patient and hold the faith. You can become more comfortable by using a combination of topical estrogen and vaginal dilators or graduated dildos. Some of you reading this might have fainted by now or can't imagine yourselves participating in what essentially amounts to a physical therapy program for your Miss Kitty. But vaginal fitness is in your future if you follow a health plan that's suited to your needs, and this usually includes continuous use of topical estrogen and gradual restretching of the vaginal tissue. It may sound unpleasant and entirely too tedious of an undertaking, but here's where humor needs to come in: imagine the shapes, sizes, and colors of dildos you can buy when embarking on this adventure. This is an example of where midlife creativity and perseverance need to be applied and where levity will be a major ingredient for success.

Estrogen isn't just involved in hot flashes, mood stability, and vaginal lubrication and elasticity. Estrogen also escorts stimulation along the central nervous system pathways. When we experience decreased estrogen with aging, stimulation with a finger, or tongue, or by rubbing against something isn't as effective as it once had been because there isn't enough estrogen to facilitate the transmission of the stimulation along the nerves. This is when lubricants and sex toys like vibrators are most helpful—but you have to be willing to use them.

Lubricants reduce friction and cool the skin, making it much nicer and more comfortable and enjoyable for us and our partners to touch our genitals. Stimulation with a vibrator adds horsepower, which compensates for the lower level of estrogen. Most women I work with who are over 50 find that using a vibrator makes it much easier to achieve orgasm as they age. Yet, I work with contemporary women all the time who still think vibrators are for whores and weirdos and are convinced that if you need a vibrator, it somehow means you love your partner less or are using the vibrator as a substitute for the one you love. There are also many women who worry that if they need a vibrator to be orgasmic, they'll get "addicted." There's no such thing as vibrator addiction or vibrator rehab. Needing to use a vibrator to be orgasmic is not a problem in and of itself. Refusing to use a vibrator to have an orgasm if you need to is a cryin' shame.

Talking to women and their partners about sex toys and lubricants can have interesting and strange effects on me and them. This is when my office shifts from counseling room to confessional and my identity from professional laity to clergy. My mention of using sex toys and other accoutrements opens the door wide for acceptance or fierce rejection of the idea. Either way, my role is to dole out hefty doses of absolution and to look for the slightest opportunity to persuade the hesitant to give sex toys a try. Explicit conversations about the specifics of sexual touching can take on a grave tone that you'd imagine using when discussing euthanizing a beloved pet but not mind-blowing orgasms. When it comes to real-life sexual issues for midlife women, too much seriousness is sure to backfire. You have to have a fair amount of resilience and levity as you're pulling out the lube and vibrator and hoping for the best—for you and your partner. Invariably, the lube bottle gets clogged, you squeeze hard, and the stuff goes all over your sheets, creating a cold, wet spot for you to lie on when your intention is to relax and have fun. Or, you have to get up and put new batteries in your vibrator, only to find you don't have any in the hardware drawer after all. If you have a male partner and are not a "cougar," chances are you may both be disappointed with his erection. My personal favorite is when my knee goes out and I have to use all sorts of special pillow arrangements just to be comfortable doing absolutely nothing: "Wait dear, let me get the bolster under my right knee"—very sexy, eh? Murphy's Law is sometimes alive and well when it comes to sex in midlife. Add this to your anachronistic reference point about how we should behave as sexually active people and you'll see that it's a miracle anyone has sex at all after 50.

Imagination, originality, and determination will ultimately lead to a more fluid definition of how you have and define sex as your body ages and your preferences and capabilities shift. In addition, you have to be willing to accept that sometimes sex is better for one partner than the other and that this is fundamentally okay. Asynchronous sexual satisfaction is par for the course as we get older. One of you might be rested while the other isn't. Or, you may be having terrific fantasies that are feeding your enthusiasm while your partner is a B-flat and can't think of anything erotic. This is normal, fine, and to be expected. When you have sex next time, things will be different and you can make up for lost experience.

It's Been Dead in the Bed for *Way* Too Long

Before many women hit midlife and are fully immersed in professional advancement and child raising, tolerating

C–minus sex as a steady diet is easier than when they hit the half-century mark and realize that lukewarm sex is all they'll ever have. When you're distracted by professional and parenting responsibilities it's much easier to let all sorts of dissatisfactions slide and go on assuming that somehow, someway, this will magically correct itself. Consider this story from one of my clients:

> My husband is a doll, but sex is a dead end with him. I have tried to spice things up, but he's got all sorts of rigid ideas about what people should do and how we should have sex. The predictability of our sex life is boring, so having sex with him doesn't interest me. It's a good thing I have my job and the kids to keep me busy and occupied. Sometimes I wonder why we got married since he's always been like this, but I love him and he is a wonderful man. I knew he would make a great father and isn't the type to have an affair, and those things are really important to me. It's hard for me to hear myself say these things about him. I feel mean—as if I am dismissing all the good about him—but I can't help it and that's what I came to see you for, right? I don't know what to do about this. The chemistry was never really there, but I am sure we can work on this and improve it. After all, we really do love one another and he would do anything for me. —Michelle, 40

This woman clearly wants her sex life with her husband to improve. But, the terror that she might end up living this way for the rest of her life is absent. Her story is missing a sense of urgency that I often hear from older women who have been living with the sexual doldrums for their entire married lives. In contrast, a midlife woman who is now more focused on her own satisfaction and fulfillment and feels her biological clock ticking has a distinctly audible parenthetical digression: "I have to get myself out of this, somehow!" Or, she will openly state something like this: "I just can't stand it anymore. I can't die without having had great sex. I love my husband, but the sex has never been good and I can't take it anymore—what should I do?" Oh, to have a magic wand—wizard, where are you?

Women can feel intense, sometimes unbearable pressure when they imagine facing the last half of their lives without ever having mind-blowing, James Bond sex before they die. This is simply unacceptable for some, and I can't say that I blame them. A voice inside them pops out and says, "Listen to me. You can't let this happen to you." If a couple has no reference point of great and satisfying sex in their sexual history, not even in the beginning when they were obsessed with one another, then she and I have a big problem on our hands—and so does her partner.

The idea of coupling with someone you don't have great sex with may seem like something that happens to women rarely, but this is not the case. There are many women who chose their mates for reasons that have absolutely nothing to do with sex: they're best friends, their partner is crazy about them and is very devoted to them, they're emotionally stable and have no wild-card tendencies, everyone else thinks they make a great pair, and her biological clock is ticking. This last factor, a ticking biological clock, is akin to that of the crocodile closing in on Captain Hook: even the boldest, bravest pirates can feel afraid, and when this is the case, a woman will sometimes marry the most stable person she sees who expresses interest and whom she likes. But when sexual chemistry is absent from the beginning, finding it as time goes by is unlikely.

As a practicing midwife and advocate of having children in your 20s or early 30s at the latest, I completely understand this and am sympathetic to women who make this choice at the figurative last minute. If they review any evolutionary biology text, they'll be able to understand why they made the decision they did. We are born with the innate and instinctual programming to reproduce and pass on our genes. And for some of us, the desire to have a child is indescribably strong and will drive us to do all sorts of things. However, if you recognize yourself in this scenario, it's highly likely that somewhere down the road you too will be a whirling dervish of frustration over your mate and sex life and be thrashing around in my office desperate to find a cure.

The reasons a couple may be sexually mismatched from the get-go are many: one partner may be more sexually experienced and sophisticated than the other; they may have different fluency levels with the language of affection and touch or differences in sexual style and willingness to be adventurous; or one party might evaluate sex based on frequency of intercourse or orgasm rather than simply enjoying it for the pleasure it provides. And let's not forget about a simple—but not so simple—lack of chemistry. When women hit midlife and are facing the prospect of a lifetime of sexual hunger and wanting, it sets off their sex alarms— as it rightly should. The problem now is, where do you go from here? Women in these situations often love their partners but have never had great sex with them. They're often not as physically attracted to their mates as would be ideal, either. Consider this story from one of my clients who was in the throes of this exact situation:

> I adore my husband and he loves me so much. Frankly, we would do anything for each other and we have a wonderful family life. But sexually, he is just not

the kind of lover I want or need. He never has been, even when we were first together. When we try to talk about changes I'd like, he gets so offended and hurt that nothing changes. I don't really want to have sex with him, and I am tired of trying to figure this out. I love him. I really do, but I am not really attracted to him. I married him because he is the sweetest, most generous, and loving man I have ever met and I knew he would be loyal and a good father. I don't know what to do. —*Sonia, 48*

This is a big problem. This story is an example of what I refer to as *marrying the family dog.* Like a well-bred golden retriever, this woman's mate is handsome (or cute), has a great personality and a sweet disposition, is terrific with kids, is easygoing, and, most important, will not stray from the yard. Her parents and friends really like him and think they make a great pair. With a description like that, it's easy to see why marrying the family dog is neither uncommon nor a bad idea in the moment. I am sure plenty of you reading this can relate to this story personally or know someone whose mate fits this description. These are perfect family-man qualities, but not necessarily the qualities of a satisfying lover.

There is no easy solution in these cases. Some women have affairs, some accept sexless marriages, and others do their best to create a noninvasive, don't-hurt-his-feelings tutorial program in the hopes that it will transform their unsatisfying partner into a real Casanova. But this is a bit like putting a Doberman costume on a golden retriever. He (or she) either *is* the breed a woman likes or isn't. Furthermore, faking that you're enjoying having sex with someone you're not really even attracted to because you don't want to hurt their feelings ends up being corrosive to the relationship and a real burden that eventually backfires, leaving a couple with a bigger mess than when they started. These conditions are torturous, and leaving them behind in the name of following what your heart and body have always desired is something I have seen midlife women have the courage and fortitude to do more often than not. The women I have worked with who have made this choice tell me they do this because they can't live an inauthentic life any longer and they're running out of time.

I am sure there are those of you who can't imagine doing such a thing to a partner who has been true, loving, supportive, and a great co-parent. I understand feeling this way. I felt the same way—until I became a sexuality counselor and heard the stories of midlife women who all said the same thing: "No matter what I ask for, he/she doesn't follow through. I can't fake it anymore—I deserve to be sexually satisfied and I am not willing to die without having had a more sexually satisfying life." Leaving your longtime mate may not be your only option, but option B will take courage and spunk and a willingness to try something entirely new and different.

Believe it or not, there are sex tutorial programs and sex coaches who couples can take advantage of when sex is dissatisfying or when they want to make good sex great. The problem here is that a partner's unwillingness to break the mold of entrenched sexual habits often tends to be part of the problem in the first place. Therefore, introducing the idea of attending an evening or weekend workshop or working with a sex coach for a while might lead to a huge fight or stall out altogether.

Keep in mind that I'm not recommending marriage counseling here. Your marriage may not be the problem; it's your sex life that's in crisis. The kind of therapy I'm talking about focuses on helping you improve your physical skills, and this often happens in the buff, in front of people you don't know. In my experience, the people who agree to this are either adventurous types who are open to new things or flat-out desperate. Either way, if you're willing to and if you can convince your partner of the potential advantage of seeing an expert who will, literally, teach you more effective and satisfying ways of having sex, then congratulations!

Remember my friend Eric, who talked about the sexiness of full-figured women? Well, he's one such expert and he's excellent at his craft (not just anyone can do this, you know).[8] Eric and other sex coaches instruct and support couples both in and out of the bedroom to maximize their pleasure by helping them perfect their actual touching skills. This may sound crazy, but the fact is there are plenty of people in the world who are blundering lovers and have no idea of how to use their hands, mouths, or other parts of their bodies in ways that really feel good and leave their lover hungering for more. The number of clients who have told me that they feel as though they're getting it on with an inexperienced teenage boy, a football coach who has only the finish line in mind, or an intercourse-focused one-celled amoeba is shockingly high.

Many people have no idea of how to explore the vast landscape of the human body and, instead, have specifically delineated landing strips when it comes to sex: the breasts and pelvis—period. And please, don't make me recount the number of bad kissers there are out there. This latter category is one that can make women both suicidal and homicidal after years of attempted correction. The idea of meeting with a stranger who is there specifically to help you have better sex may feel unimaginable and out of the question. But if the alternative is an affair, separation, or divorce, advice from a skilled craftsperson may be just what you need. When you think about it, if you grew up in a family where touching and being touched was in short order, how would you have learned how to touch in a way that was intuitive or comfortable for both of you? Touch is a language unto itself, and like any other language, fluency is best acquired in childhood, when your brain is most flexible and receptive and when you have less inhibition. Learning how to touch later in life is not impossible, but it can be very difficult. I realize that for some people, asking for specific instruction for improved sex or even going the next step and demonstrating your existing skill set may feel impossible. But, if better sex is what you're after, then go to someone who specializes in helping people learn how to have it and just jump in with both feet. I guarantee you won't be their first customer.

Sex is a strong, primal desire that many of us don't imagine women hunger for, or even should want so badly that they would turn their lives upside down when everything but sex is tidy and well placed.

Whether a woman married the family dog or is struggling with sexual dissatisfaction and her partner won't participate in efforts to make things better, when this has been the case for years, it's the mature woman in her Decade of Hell who's most likely to slay this dragon and find a new kingdom to reside in. Children are grown and in college, her professional life is coasting or may be on the rise, and she decides she cannot waste a precious moment of whatever time she has left. There's no guarantee that she might succeed in her mission to find what fulfills the dreams she has created for herself or to find exactly what she's looking for. Nonetheless, she chooses not to hang around in the same place any longer, hoping things will get better after a long time of trying.

In some cases, women simply cannot manage the upheaval of leaving a long-term marriage when everything but sex falls under the category of "just fine" or "really comfortable." This is a deeply personal decision that each person has to make. I would never fault someone for making an honest and seriously considered choice after weighing all the alternatives available. In the end, you will be the one who lives with whatever choice you make. However, I encourage you to review all your options—sex coaching included—before you stay wedded to a lifetime of sexual unhappiness.

To Sum It All Up

The most important aspects of pleasure for midlife women and the sense of power they give us are that we have to work smarter and more creatively to keep our markers of emotional well-being intact. And when we do, the payoff can be mighty sweet. There is something deeply liberating about finally being able to release some expectations we have of ourselves, others, and life in general while also orchestrating accomplishments and discoveries we've always hoped for and are really attainable. For women who have always looked at midlife and aging as terrifying prospects, the beginning of the end of good and easy living, or the point at which sex runs cold forevermore, I recommend you reconsider this. Frankly, there's nothing quite like looking at the last 30 years or so of essentially uncomplicated living (with luck) to spur you in the right direction and force you to do what you've always wanted to do. As I see it in my own life and in those of other women, we're granted an amazing opportunity after more or less a half century of living to make great things happen in life—if we choose to do so. Put down your grief, your despair, and your sense of doom and get a piece of paper and a pencil. Start your bucket list and think and dream big. There's no time like the present, and frankly, it's what you have most in your favor.

QUESTIONS TO ASK YOURSELF

1. What are my honest feelings about myself as a middle-aged woman and about middle age in general?

2. Have I "let myself go" in midlife? If so, how has this affected my sense of being powerful in the world and accessing pleasure?

3. Am I willing to shore up my markers of emotional well-being so I'll then be able to access pleasure and feel better about life and sex in general? If not, why?

4. Do my partner and I have a reference point in our history as a couple for having experienced great sex? If not, why have I stayed in a relationship that has never been sexually satisfying for me? How important is sex to me?

5. What are my ideas of how midlife women are supposed to behave sexually, and where did these ideas come from?

6. Do I know any midlife women who embody and demonstrate a kind of living and sexuality

that I find appealing and desirable? What is it specifically about them that makes me see them this way?

7. What was my mother like as a midlife woman? What example did she set regarding sexuality at midlife? Was it positive or negative, and how much of this did I assume or reject?

8. What things would I like to experience sexually that my partner flatly opposes? If there are some, what's my plan for managing this disappointment?

9. On a scale of one to ten, how would I rate my sense of humor and levity when it comes to sex and not having things go exactly as I planned? Do I think sex should always be taken very seriously, or can I have a light attitude about it?

10. How wedded am I to the idea that both my partner and I should be equally satisfied when we have sex? Can I easily, comfortably accept that sometimes it's better for one of us than it is for the other?

11. How open am I to using sex toys and other sexual aids or consulting a sex coach? If I am not open to it, why? How about my partner?

12. Have I ever considered leaving my relationship because I feel sexually dissatisfied so much of the time? If so and I haven't left, what's keeping me there, and am I willing to risk living for the rest of my life as a sexually dissatisfied person?

13. Do I have a good gynecological health-care provider who I am willing to talk honestly with about genital health problems I may be having that are interfering with having comfortable sex? If not, am I willing to see someone else?

CHAPTER 6

HONESTLY, IT'S ALL HE THINKS ABOUT

*Part of the reason that men seem so much
less loving than women is that men's behavior
is measured with a feminine ruler.*

—FRANCESCA M. CANCIAN

Over the past few years, men's sexual desires and appetites have made big headlines in the news. The stories of high-profile philanderers and the fallout from their behavior have read like raunchy and exaggerated tabloid exposés, but the stories are true. Former New York governor and attorney general Eliot Spitzer, former North Carolina senator John Edwards, Tiger Woods, and former California

governor Arnold Schwarzenegger have added great di-
mension to the definition of *slimeball* while simultaneously
catapulting their emotionally stunned and ravaged wives
into public heroines. This unseemly and tasteless behavior
has left many of us wondering the same thing: *what is it
with men?* We rarely see women making these sorts of er-
rors, and when a woman does step over the line—Monica
Lewinsky style—folks are reticent to forgive and forget.
When women's sexual exploits land them in the limelight,
they're deemed trashy, stupid whores. Men on the other
hand—well, what do you expect? They're just acting like
men.

Many of the women I work with complain that their
own partner's sexual desire is bigger than life, or at least
much bigger than theirs. These women experience every
gesture, affectionate touch, and sometimes conversation
as a sexual advance and as a result, they develop strategies to minimize contact with their partners (even when
they love and are attracted to them) so as not to encourage them or give them "any ideas" that they're interested
in sex. When this dynamic takes hold, women repeatedly
invent reasons why having sex is not an option while rag-
ing about their partners' insatiable appetites. Anger then
becomes the most pervasive and operant emotion for both
partners: she's angry because she always feels stalked and
he because she is completely unavailable and critical. Despite pervasive assumptions that as a culture we've become
more sexually sophisticated and active (as evidenced by our
feeding frenzy over the *Fifty Shades Trilogy*), most couples
are not having sex as often as many men would like to or
others think they are. The destructive impact of disparate
sexual appetites often goes unaddressed until a catastro-
phe, like severe estrangement or an affair—that either he or

she is having—destabilizes the relationship. Based on many conversations I have had with men about sex, it seems that they really do look at sex differently. At the risk of sounding crude beyond repair, men can more easily accept sex as an important bodily function that will put someone or something—like their marriage—at risk if ignored for too long. And even though the women they love find it hard to believe at times, they are selective about whom they want to experience this bodily function with. Men who love their women partners want to have sex with them—not just anyone. Further, men have told me time and again that having sex with their women partners is a way for them to both express their love and feel loved in return.

There is absolutely no question that men and women approach sex differently, and much of this has to do with differences in brain function as well as hormones. Women's brains are shaped by estrogen, men's by testosterone. And whether or not you believe that a testosterone-dominant brain thinks only about sex and is shortsighted, less able to think through the consequences of behavior, and disturbingly and disappointingly nonverbal, based on the news headlines, it's easy to overgeneralize about men and the choices they make about sex. But as a sexuality counselor to many heterosexual couples, I have met plenty of men living celibate lives because their sexual advances have been shunned for months and sometimes years by their female partners. They don't seek alternative sex partners because they love their mates and don't want to betray them. Many men have demonstrated amazing tolerance for and patience with their partner's disinterest in sexual intimacy out of a combination of respect and regard and, frankly, an inability to push back when the woman they love says "No!" a thousand times over. When these men have spoken to me about their hopeless sexual lives, their voices are tired and sad. They don't understand their wives' anger and why their desire for her—and only her—is such a turnoff. Why is sex—which feels so good, important, and necessary to them—met with such negativity and resistance?

Resolution of this strife and sexual heartache depends on the couple being aware of and genuinely acknowledging the biological differences between men's and women's brains and how these differences affect behavior. Both partners need to be willing to educate themselves, communicate honestly, and then develop and implement strategies that will better allow them to meet one another's needs and desires as much as possible. This takes skill, sensitivity, and a mind open to approaching sex from a different perspective. Partners also need to be willing to accept that their desires can't always be met exactly the way they would like them to be and that this is a normal part of a monogamous sexual partnership.

BIOLOGY AND SOCIAL PRESSURES

Human sexuality is rooted in our reproductive capacity and our drive to perpetuate the species. Men's biology makes them fertile at all times and drives them unceasingly toward sex. Women's biology makes them fertile on a cyclic basis that is less reliable and often deliberately tampered with to prevent conception. This difference between daily fertility and monthly fertility and the risks sometimes associated with it is more influential than we often realize. While we have moved way beyond mere perpetuation of the species as a motive for having sex, we remain slaves to our biology to some extent.

A particular fact about gender-specific neurobiology bears mentioning at this point, not as an excuse for men's behavior but as an explanation. The area of the brain responsible for sexual pursuit in men is two and a half times bigger than that in women.[9] While biology isn't destiny and both men and women pursue sex for reasons related to relational bonding and recreation, this fact alone certainly helps us understand more about the male sex drive. This doesn't mean men should be given carte blanche to have sex anytime and with any available partner. But biological anthropologist Helen Fisher, Ph.D., who specializes in studying the human brain in love, dispels the myth that they would want to in the first place. Her article "8 Surprising Truths About Men" would cause anyone who believes that all men are after is sex to pause and reconsider their perspective on men in relationships.[10] The good news is that being aware of this makes us better informed and hopefully more compassionate toward one another. It also allows us the opportunity to make behavioral modifications that can work in our favor. This includes changing our minds and shedding our limiting ideas of what sex is for—and how, when, and why we're supposed to have it. It also helps us understand more about why men act the ways they do when it comes to pursuing their mates with sex on their minds.

The following relates an interesting and informative situation I encountered that will really help women understand how men feel during much of their lives. Although this story may seem like the opposite of men wanting sex all the time, that is exactly what this man describes his experience to have been until after the age of 60, which speaks to some of the downsides of the male sex drive, especially for men.

A healthy, attractive woman and her husband, both in their early 60s, came to see me once because the woman was concerned about her husband's decreased interest in sex. She was worried that he wasn't sexually attracted to her anymore because his interest had dropped off noticeably. He had always had a big appetite for sex and they had successfully managed and often enjoyed this for years without difficulty. This was a happily married couple and her worry and fear ran deep. When you read his response below, consider what it must really feel like to be so cognizant of your sex drive so much of the time and how demanding it can be.

> My whole life, I have always felt preoccupied by sexual thoughts and feelings. My desire was intense and was present at almost every moment. I could really have had sex just about anytime, day or night. It was always on my mind. This is the first time in my life that I actually have any brain space that allows for thinking about something other than sex for extended periods of time, and I am finding myself really enjoying it! It is a new experience for me, and my decreased interest has nothing to do with not being attracted to my wife anymore. It simply seems to be a factor of my own aging. I am perfectly healthy, don't need any medications, and don't have any illnesses or diseases. But for whatever reasons, I am not focused on sex the way I used to be and frankly, I am finding it to be a real relief. —Bob, 63

This was the most concise description I had ever heard of what it really feels like to have so much more testosterone running through you than estrogen. Whatever you believe about the research regarding how testosterone affects cognition, decision making, and perspective, it's unequivocal that a high level of testosterone can make seeking, having, and enjoying sex a somewhat urgent matter on a frequent basis. According to this man, this urgency can be downright intrusive and demanding and can impact life in ways that are limiting. Unfortunately, most women don't seem to know this about men, and men have a hard time explaining it in such a way that it elicits compassion as opposed to fury. We all know the "I just can't help it!" explanation only goes so far.

Most women I know and have worked with couldn't possibly imagine feeling this way. In complete contrast, they have needed to work diligently to reassure themselves that pleasure—especially sexual pleasure—is essentially safe, worthwhile, and good for them. As adolescents, we're trained to fear and resist our sexuality. Teen girls learn all about the risks associated with sexual activity, not the joys of having sex. Unplanned pregnancies, STIs, ruined reputations, and young boys wanting them for nothing else is the script commonly and repeatedly read to girls as their sexual energy comes into the foreground. The overall message is clear: do all you can to shun your own sexual impulses and drives, for this is the safe, ladylike, and righteous thing to do. Even women who have confidence in their sexuality and have accepted that pleasure isn't wrong can feel put upon by a male partner whose sexuality is so strongly supported by their biology and readily accepted (if not encouraged) by their families and culture.

WHAT I'M REALLY TRYING TO SAY . . .

Men would do themselves a big favor if they would at least mention to women that having sex is their way of communicating the following: I miss you, I love you, I want you, and I appreciate you and everything you do for me and our family. Men have also explained to me that they will turn to sex as a way of apologizing, resolving tensions, and reconnecting with their partners when the silent treatment is being metered out and tensions are running high. This is counterintuitive for women, and it drives them wild. At a time like that, most women would rather stab their partners than have sex with them. These are the moments when women want to talk, which is a death knell to a man who is likely to find even the thought of more conversation a sex-killer if there ever was one. In tumultuous times, plenty of men want to work through it with great thrusting, not conversation—and not just with anyone. This is the critical piece that women seem to forget or are blind to. Unless you've married a guy who could substitute for the schmucks in the headlines, you're likely to have a man in your life who wants to have sex with you and only you to make things better between the two of you. This has greater value than many women are willing to give it. And you never know, it might work to fix things up better than you think—but you have to be willing to try it.

The disparities between men's and women's appetites and expressions of desire contribute greatly to tension between couples. When the difference between their partners' experience is so antithetical to their own, many women are left struggling to remain self-assured in their sexuality. Men often do want to have sex more frequently than women, and the true meaning of their expressions of longing frequently get lost in the inevitably contentious scene at the kitchen sink, which goes something like this: Wife is washing vegetables in preparation for dinner. Husband comes up from behind and puts his arms around her waist, starts to kiss her neck, cups her breasts in his hands, and says something like "I *love* these tits—I can't get enough of them." This results in an automatic erection for him and a stiffening of her entire body because she's convinced that he wants intercourse right at that very moment. A fight ensues between them and sex is delayed for another month; she'll show him! Sound familiar? If so, join the ranks of the many women who have described this to me over the years. It's a common story, and while I understand women's irritation—after all, she is trying to wash vegetables, and women are not sex objects—I also have come to believe that women can be way too hard on their male partners. Furthermore, not every erection must be managed and relieved by the woman who inspired it. In fact, an erection can be accepted as simply that—an erection, not a call to duty.

When this is the first story I'm told by a woman who's seeking sexuality counseling, I always ask her if she can recall a time in the history of the relationship when she would have welcomed these advances and the couple's participation and desire were on an even par. Once in a while, women tell me that sex was never that great, but because of the emotional connection they felt they made the decision to couple anyway, hoping things would improve or just accepting that sex wasn't their strong suit as a couple. But the majority of women I see can easily recall sexier times with their partners, early on in the relationship, before they were married, had kids, and had big responsibilities. This makes it sound as if marriage and sustained, satisfying sex are mutually exclusive. Sadly, many people believe this and live it. But from my vantage point, I can see that things don't have to be this way. Usually when they are, something that has led a woman away from her sexuality has been going on for way too long, causing her male partner

to desperately try to chase her down in hopes of changing her mind. When this scenario is repeatedly replayed,
the anger it generates can drive a deep wedge between a
woman and a man. In order for there to be sexual harmony
in any couple with disparate sexual appetites, *both* partners need to feel comfortable with and anchored in their
own sexuality first and foremost, and this is often harder
for women than it is for men. One important piece in the
puzzle of bringing harmony and comfort is to understand
and have compassion for the man you're partnering with.
So let's delve a bit deeper into how men communicate.

MAN SPEAK

Frankly, I love men, and in part it's for the exact reason
that they make so many of their women partners angry:
they communicate feelings and opinions with greater brevity and often through their bodies, not through conversation, which is an enviable and handy trait as far as I am
concerned. This can be a refreshing approach to getting a
point across with speed and valuable accuracy. But in their
female partners it can also create an overwhelming sense
of rage and the unequivocal belief that their men are not
paying attention or don't care about how they feel or what
they have to say. Sometimes this is true. But more often
than not, it just isn't the case. Men are actually wired to
communicate in different ways and are neurologically inclined to solve problems rather than converse. Because love
and emotion are shown through physical actions versus
nurturing conversations, men often shut down when their
wives or partners start repeating themselves in a conversation. They just can't tolerate it, which, of course, leads their

partners to assume they're not listening at all. A man's somatic way of communicating his attachment to the people and things he cares about may be different, but it isn't inferior to a woman's method. Plus, in some situations it has tremendous appeal and value.

When Hurricane Irene hit the Northeast in August of 2011, the county I live in in western Massachusetts was one of the two hardest hit. By late morning, my partner and I were forced to evacuate our home because water was bounding down the mountainside that abuts our property, putting our house's foundation in danger and threatening to cut off access on our road. The flow of water had reached a record height and speed. I had never seen anything like it. If not for the men in our town, we would have been sunk— literally. One man in particular, my friend Mike, exemplifies what I am talking about.

Mike has a company whose motto is "No Job Too Odd." This is the absolute truth. Mike does everything from cleaning out fish tanks to excavating with a bulldozer, and often in the same day. And while Mike is a savvy businessman, I have also never known anyone so generous and kind about sharing the skills he has with those in need, business aside. He may not leap at the opportunity to help you process your feelings about whatever problem it is he's solving for you, but he'll do anything and everything he can to minimize its impact on your life and psyche. Conversations are great, but they have their limitations. When Hurricane Irene seemed to be dismantling the world—mine included— Mike showed up, as always, to pump the five feet of water out of our cellar, deal with the smell of gasoline that was emanating from our basement, and make sure we didn't drown, explode, or get electrocuted. This sort of hands-on, get-the-job-done approach is Mike's way of showing us that our friendship goes both ways. I bring him home-made granola and tell him every time I see him that he's one of my best friends. In turn he rescues me from many of life's unexpected burdens that I simply have no idea how to lessen or resolve. As I watched the orchestrated efforts made by Mike and other men involved in our rescue, I realized that my life is made all the better by men—they help me with tasks my female brain and musculature can't manage easily and with getting to the heart of a matter. Men may be less comfortable with and fluent when expressing their feelings through words, but make no mistake about it, every one of the men who helped us during and after the storm cared deeply about our safety and welfare.

So if you're feeling frustrated with your man, take a step back and look at his actions. If you remember that he communicates not through words but through his physicality, you're likely to feel more compassionate toward his needs. You'll also be better able to feel secure in yourself when you realize that not every sexual advance is a need for sexual satisfaction; rather, it's just your man saying that he loves you. You can turn down his advances if you're truly not in the mood, but don't misinterpret them and don't shame him for having them. Don't think that your man looks at you and only wants you for sex or that he doesn't appreciate everything you do. Thinking this way will just lead to anger or guilt and eventually harm your sexual relationship even more. If you want to find your way back to your man, try moving into your own body more and do something with him that's physical but not necessarily sexual. Ride your bikes together, take a hike, work on a house project. Communication is a two-way street, and both members of a relationship need to have at least an intermediate level of knowledge about each other's dialects in order to get your points across. You don't have to be a certified translator, but the ability to convey your thoughts and feelings certainly makes for more successful and satisfying communication. Remember, talking is not the only way to get a point across. Sometimes, the act of doing something can leave a clearer, more lasting impression as a way to express how you feel.

How Can Women Say "Yes" More Often, "No" When They Really Mean It, AND Stay Self-Assured?

In order for women to feel more respectful and appreciative of men's sexuality, they must make better friends with their own. This is directly linked to the thesis of this book, pleasure begets pleasure, and sexual pleasure is no exception to this. In turn, pleasure enhances self-empowerment, which includes feeling self-assured and resilient, even where sexuality is concerned.

When women come to see me for sexuality counseling with the chief complaint that they have no time for sex or that all their husband wants is sex, more often than not I ask them, "What *exactly* do you expend energy on that makes having sex feel like climbing Everest?" Generally speaking, women look at me with an air of both curiosity and indignation, as if simply because I am another working-woman, I would know the answer to this question.

For women, choosing a life filled with pleasure means engaging in a wrestling match between how they think they should be in the world and how they feel best. This often means a serious appraisal of our self-worth and a re-assurance that we have innate goodness—even if we're not helping everyone else. This is not a quandary men regularly find themselves in, but it's very common for women.

In general, it doesn't seem as difficult for men to make the choice to grant space for pleasure and sex as it is for women, which pisses us off to no end. In the absence of an anxiety disorder or other psychological malady, men seem more able to let go of the *shoulds* and focus on what's actually happening and possible in the moment. When men have described their decision-making processes to me, they have seemed less focused on possible consequences and forecasting potential disasters. And while this may be somewhat shortsighted and has gotten some men in big trouble, there is a liberating quality to it. And maybe biology does have something to do with this. But barring blatant recklessness and weak moral character, this in-the-moment way of thinking and acting can make life sweeter and sexual energy and satisfaction easier to enjoy more often.

Listening to heterosexual women complain in exasperated tones about how frustrating it is to have a partner who doesn't communicate about how he feels has taught me that human beings are at a high risk of misinterpreting information when they look at it through a gender-specific lens. During women's tearful stories about how frustrated they are with their seemingly sexually deranged husbands chasing after them *all the time,* I often am thinking, *He's communicating, just not through the spoken word.*

The most blatant example of this occurred during a session with a couple who were struggling terribly and whose sex life had been virtually absent for a few years. He was a talented surgeon in great demand in his specialty, they had children, and she was a stay-at-home mother. She had been complaining in the session about how he was so absent from their family and did nothing on behalf of all of them, yet he still wanted to have sex. It was then that I pointed out to her that he was doing quite a bit for their family by working such long hours and supporting all of them without ever questioning his role or dedication to doing so. This took her by surprise and was an obvious comfort to him. She had never considered that his attachment, love, and desire to have his family were being expressed through his actions. She had never really asked him how he felt about his work and took it for granted that this was his role—whether it was suiting him or not didn't seem relevant to her. And yes, there was fine-tuning to be done here and a compromise needed to be struck between her needs and his. But, her exasperated description of his not doing anything for them was a hurtful and gross overstatement that resulted in her filibustering his idea to have sex sometimes. That guy didn't stand a chance of getting laid under these circumstances.

WOMEN'S WAYS AREN'T ALWAYS BETTER

I have had intimate relationships with men that have been very satisfying to me both emotionally and sexually. And, at the risk of sounding trite, some of my best friends are men. But now that I'm in a same-sex marriage, the world identifies me as a lesbian while I consider myself to be a bisexual woman who landed on the same-sex-partner side of love. It just so happens that I fell head over heels for a woman. Nothing political about it, simply fate.

Like all happily wedded couples, we have our moments when frustration reigns and when there are things about each of us that are hard for the other to take. The number one irritant for me is that my partner perseverates in conversations—like women are notorious for doing. Or, as one of my male clients put it, "Why do women repeat the same things at least three times in every conversation? If she tells me once, that's really enough; I've got it." When my partner does this over the course of a day or a week, there is invariably trouble in paradise. These are times when I will literally tell her to "man up and stop talking so much." If you think women do the conversation thing just right, think again. When we first got involved, I really wasn't sure of our lasting potential because of this. I had talking head-aches on a regular basis, and I was so tired from the daily review of how I felt and then how she felt that I started to shut down altogether . . . just like women tell me men do. Perhaps this is why I have such compassion for them. I know how it feels to have someone talk your ear off and expect you to give back in the same way—whether you can, want to, or are up to it is irrelevant. *And* there is this astoundingly unrelenting assumption that communicating this way is the *right* and *best* way to express what's on your mind. Never mind that I thought my actions spoke louder than words. My partner wanted words and lots of them. If I grabbed an opportunity for a brief respite and to try and catch my breath, I would risk having her question me about whether or not I was holding back, unwilling to express myself, or maybe not wanting to meet her emotional needs. Unlike most men I know, who use a few words to get their points across and then move along, my partner and I—because we're women—have a propensity for complex, labyrinthine, and lengthy conversations about things I know I could tidy up with a man in relatively short order. I once asked my friend Mike if he was mad at me about something because I hadn't heard from him all week. His response: "No, if I were mad at you, I would have told you."

End of discussion, nothing more to say. Women often think that men's brevity and laconic tendencies reflect a lack of personal depth, serious consideration of the topic, or capacity for insight. Not necessarily. It's simply an abbreviated way of expressing oneself verbally that comes naturally to men, and many women find that very difficult to relate to, if not worthy of suspicion.

Women who find themselves frustrated with their male partners for what they're not talking about need to remember that speaking is but one form of communicating thoughts and feelings. And, how about making more of an effort to learn men's dialect instead of holding it against them and refusing to have sex with them because they won't talk more? But you can't do this without feeling assured in your own sexuality as a valid and creative form of communication. This takes dedicated practice, devotion to a life filled with pleasure, and the belief that having sex is a way to express feelings of all sorts, including love, devotion, and attachment, but not the only way. For some, sexual engagement is a fine way to mend fences, express creativity, and relieve stress and tension. In my opinion and experience, there isn't anything wrong with this but it's more often a man's way than a woman's. I don't assume for a moment that the communication gap between men and women could be easily bridged if only women would be more compassionate about men's biology and the way it shapes their sex drives. If you are struggling with a male partner, explore how comfortable you are with your own sexuality and sex in general. Also, if you feel estranged from sex, keep asking yourself whether or not your estrangement is connected to your unwillingness to welcome pleasure into your life daily and if your partner has a different relationship with pleasurable living than you do. This is worthy

WOMEN, SEX, POWER & PLEASURE

of pondering for both of your sakes and in the interest of improving harmony in your relationship.

QUESTIONS TO ASK YOURSELF

1. Am I willing to lie next to my partner while he takes responsibility for self-pleasuring if I don't want to have sex? If I'm not, why? If I am, am I able to do this without judging him for his desire?

2. Name the ways your male partner expresses his attachment to you that are not sexual and ask yourself, *do I express my appreciation of these in return, and if so, how?*

3. Do I feel it's wrong for my partner to want sex as a way of my showing my appreciation for him? If so, why, and how might I see it differently after reading this chapter?

4. Have I ever thought that sex is a way of communicating more than loving devotion and sexual arousal? If not, why, and am I willing to be persuaded otherwise?

5. What is it about my male partner that attracts me sexually? If these things are still present and we haven't been having sex, why not? What are the obstacles?

6. Does the idea of sex as a necessary bodily function offend me? If so, what can I do about this to lessen my negative thinking and response?

7. Am I willing to learn more about how men's brains actually work so I can better understand the differences between us?

CHAPTER 7

BECOMING YOUR OWN ACTIVIST

*Nobody could deny the intellectual flexibility
of our species, and nobody could deny that culture
can shape and structure human pleasure.*

—PAUL BLOOM

The impact of one's culture on their overall worldview should never be forgotten or underestimated. I keep this in mind every time I work with someone as a sexuality counselor or a midwife and when I am personally struggling to find my way out of a vexing situation. Our ethnicity and cultural orientation shape and influence our development and decision-making processes throughout life, whether we're conscious of it or not. This is especially complicated for people who have their feet in two very different worlds—one inside the home of their family of origin and one on the other side of the front door.

I grew up in a bilingual, bicultural Greek home smack in the middle of Midwest America. There are some things about me that are straight out of the cherry capital of the USA: I am friendly, make conversation easily, and would be the first one to bring a new neighbor a welcoming casserole. But, when it comes to my psyche and greater worldview, my mother's ethnicity and Hellenic heritage are predominantly responsible for shaping my perspectives on life, pleasure, and sexuality. There is no question that I am more a Greek than I am a midwesterner—like it or not, for better and for worse.

Greeks are loud, opinionated, pushy, domineering, belittling of non-Greeks, grudge holders for a lifetime, highly critical of others, and indulgent of their sons while unrelentingly strict with their daughters. They can also be obnoxiously exclusive and ethnocentric to the point of cruelty. On the other hand, Greeks are fabulous orators, passionate about life, masters of simple fare, friendly, willing to embrace fate gracefully, mystical, they mourn their dead in beautiful and healthy ways, and, above and beyond all else, celebrate life's pleasures often and without hesitation. This last trait is what I am most grateful to have inherited from the Greek side of my family. This is also what has most informed and influenced the thesis of this book and my way of living. Greeks are the progenitors of ancient civilization *and* pleasurable living. Without the latter, we wouldn't be Greeks.

Raising bilingual and bicultural children was not in fashion in the 1960s, and my parents endured plenty of criticism from American and Greek friends who thought it unnecessary, backward, and a bit pedantic. But, they were ahead of their time, and because of my mother's assumed ethnic dominance and the absence of my father's family, my father learned Greek to unify our family linguistically and adopted my mother's cultural practices. One such practice—*kambanyatico*—is an example of one of the many rituals I witnessed and enjoyed that were constant reminders of the importance and value of partaking in life's simple pleasures as often as possible.

Kambanyatico is a colloquial term that originated on the island of Patmos, where my maternal grandmother is from. It is a break taken in the late afternoon that is initiated by the ringing of the *kambana,* or bells, in the Monastery of Saint John the Divine, which gives the island its notoriety and status as holy ground. Whenever the day allowed for it, everything in our household stopped at about 3 P.M. so my grandmother and mother could regroup and have coffee, biscuits, feta, and plenty of conversation. I remember the *brika* used to make the coffee, the decorative cups it was poured into, the traditional *koolourikia* biscuits my grandmother made, and the array of topics covered in the half hour or so that they would spend together. Fast-forward 45 years and kambanyatico is alive and well in my own home, and it's just as restorative and important to me as it had been to them. While I am not a fan of Turkish coffee and have yet to inherit those beautiful cups, my own version of this afternoon sacrament is well cemented in my life, including the koolourikia, which I now make myself. Kambanyatico is not just a coffee break. It is an example of the many pleasurable things I do often that keep me attuned to my senses and eventually feed into my sexuality.

I am sure some of you are struggling to make the leap from kambanyatico to keeping yourself sexually engaged. Fair enough. But move beyond the simple ritual to the implied message: coffee is delicious and so are biscuits and feta. Take time to sit down and fully enjoy them in the company of someone you care for, and let the pleasure of doing so inform and influence you. Don't let the chores and responsibilities of the day keep you from the pleasures life has to offer. Think of this comparatively; kambanyatico is miles away from drinking a latte from a paper cup while you're driving to your next appointment and talking on your cell phone. The ingredients may be the same, but the experiences couldn't be more diametrically opposed.

SWIMMING AGAINST THE TIDE
OF THE ANTIPLEASURE CULTURE

Contemporary American culture has turned multitasking, blind repetition, and virtual contact into great American pastimes. I have witnessed people of all ages attempting with zeal and disturbing determination to do so many things simultaneously that it makes me fear for their lives and mine. The necessity of passing legislation that makes talking and texting while driving crimes indicates just how addictive and problematic multitasking can be—enough that lawmakers needed to intervene.

In my medical office, we have signs everywhere that say, PLEASE, TURN OFF YOUR CELL PHONE. And yet, ringtones continue to be heard throughout our office, exam rooms included. Talking on a cell phone or texting while doing just about everything else—including while your health care provider is doing your Pap smear—reveals just how habituated so many of us have become to multitasking in oblivion. This last example is not something I made up—it really happened to me in my office. When I confronted my patient, she was honestly confounded by my ire. I left my visit with her feeling utterly depersonalized. I could have been a chimp doing her Pap smear, and I am not convinced she would have noticed.

Cell phones and other ubiquitous communication devices are terrific and handy inventions. But our polyamorous relationships with them have impaired our ability to fully focus on communicating in real time with real people, including the ones we have sex with. Doing two (or more) things at once can't help but detract from our experiences of each since it's difficult to fully attend to anything when your attention is divided, especially as we age. The phrase *come to your senses* has never been more apropos or potentially lifesaving (and relationship rescuing) than at present. Technological advancements designed to accelerate and increase communication between people for personal or professional reasons represent the best of human ingenuity. But they've proven to have a big downside. The virtual and somewhat automated communication they grant us and its direct connection and contribution to multitasking have exacerbated what I refer to as *sensual atrophy syndrome* (SAS), which is a marked estrangement from life's pleasures. In part, this comes from a bold resistance to prioritizing communicating with others while giving them your undivided attention. SAS undermines the pleasure-begets-pleasure model that feeds emotional well-being, empowered living, and easier access to our sexuality.

More and more often in my sexuality counseling practice, I am trying to help individuals and couples manage the impact of technological advancements and devices on their intimate and personal lives. I had one couple who had reached a true crisis point when the husband's love of his BlackBerry had, evidently, exceeded the love he felt for his wife. She was convinced of this when she discovered that he had slid his BlackBerry under the mattress on his side of the bed in such a way that it was visible during intercourse in the missionary position. Needless to say, this couple's marriage was in major trouble. I realize this example is extreme, but there are plenty more out there that are close to that. Laptops, iPads, and BlackBerrys are littering bedrooms across America and causing all sorts of marital rifts, not to mention sleep problems. There's nothing more damaging to any relationship than feeling as though you *never* have the person's undivided attention. In relationships that include sex, it's the biggest anti-aphrodisiac I know of.

MIXING THE OLD WITH THE NEW

Interspersing familiar, new, and different pleasurable activities throughout your day and giving them your undivided attention is the best way I know of to vanquish SAS or prevent it in the first place. No matter what demands lie before you, there is always a way to participate in pleasurable activities provided that you prioritize them and separate them from your work. Think of it as regular exercise to combat SAS. Doing so helps you stay limber and more capable of moving into the slipstream of your sexuality with greater ease and confidence. When people tell me they have no sexual interest or desire, the first thing I want to know is how they live their lives. If their answer describes a life jam-packed with chores or a highly repetitive, choreographed, and memorized script of activities along with little time spent doing pleasurable things, this is where my sexuality counseling will begin.

Our libidos are cultivated and nurtured by living fully engaged and ever-changing sensual lives. Like all other disciplined practices—eating and sleeping well, exercising—you need to pay attention to it for the rest of your life and to fine-tune your approach in order to maximize the benefits.

Diversifying your pleasurable activities regularly helps to avoid the deadening impact of repetition, which negatively impacts efforts to stay awake and engaged in the long run. There is a delicate balance to be struck here between the pleasure we receive from known and comforting practices versus the pleasure and *activation* we receive from things that are new and different. Kambanyatico is a wonderful break—but my work life doesn't allow me to enjoy it at home every day. Sometimes I experience its benefits in a new coffee shop with a friend or colleague, and the newness combined with the comforts of the known can make kambanyatico outside of my home even more satisfying.

Optimally, the pleasure we experience should run on a continuum with *sedate* on one end and *near-death* on the other. Living exclusively to the left or the right of the apex of the bell curve is just as dangerous as remaining at the apex of average. Search for things that are mildly tantalizing while regularly scanning the horizon for something that could blow your mind. There is undeniable pleasure and benefit in the calming effects of an evening bath, just as there is in an orgasm so intense that your life flashes before you and you think you might die from it—and don't really mind if you do. The panoply of pleasurable stimuli in our lives should feel and be vast, broad, and indefinite. And while this is sometimes hard to pull off in the face of the demands of daily life, it is by no means impossible. You just have to work at it. Otherwise, it won't be only sexual ennui and decreased libido you'll be suffering from. Sooner or later, just about everything takes on the feel and look of an open prairie: flat as a pancake—no rolling hills, no valleys, no differences that pique your curiosity. Sameness—day in and day out—makes us duds in our daily lives and sexually. It also has an undeniably disempowering effect. When a woman comes to me and tells me she's still attracted to her partner and enjoys sex when they have it, but for some inexplicable reason it's a sexual dead zone at home, I always ask how things go when they're on vacation. If she says, "Oh, we always have sex on vacation," chances are that their day-to-day lives are bone dry and have made them dull and insensitive to everything, including one another. Give them just a weekend away (or even 36 hours—remember the 4 or 6 x 36 rule?) in a new and different place that stimulates their senses with things they've never seen, heard, smelled, or touched and they'll transform into hotties in no time. Plenty of people haven't changed their daily routines in months or years. This is dangerous living and can easily result in shattering boredom without our realizing it until crisis hits. But few people make the connection between how their approach to life impacts their sense of feeling powerful and their appetite for and experience of sex.

As I write this, I too am reminded of the deadliness of repetition and the status quo. My partner and I have made the decision to live simpler, less costly lives. This has meant forfeiting a certain amount of travel and we rarely eat out. But neither greater simplicity nor conscious spending should dictate or determine all our menus and new experiences. Nonetheless, as middle-aged rural dwellers we commute to work, are exhausted at the end of our workdays, and fall into the high-risk category for the sexual doldrums. We're often in our pajamas by 7 P.M., scanning the television menu for our shows, and we are experts at talking ourselves out of going anywhere so we don't have to drive. This has had some very deleterious effects.

Becoming a bore or a dolt and simply acquiescing to low-effort activities, meals, or even outfits is not uncommon, especially as we age. Loss of stamina, aches and pains, and a longing for simplifying our often complicated worlds can transform even the once very spunky and adventurous individual into the kind of aging person they loathed in their 20s and swore they would never become. No doubt some of you know exactly what I mean.

The power and influence of stimulating our senses in new and different ways should never be underestimated or avoided. Even something as simple as a new brassiere can change your partner's typical reaction in the bedroom. Many of us look for what's affordable and will successfully keep "the girls" up and in line, but the alluring effect of a new and revealing bra can never be overstated. In fact, just the right new bra can have nothing short of the Lazarus effect on you and your partner and raise you both from the figurative dead. You could go from desultory, mindless C-minus to hot and steamy for under a hundred dollars. Who cares if it's comfortable or offers great support? Just buy the thing and see what happens!

Contrary to assumption and popular belief, there is no such thing as spontaneous, effortless sex. This is especially true as we age and experience the physical wear and tear of growing older. You need to be doing preparatory work for sex every day if you want to keep it in the foreground of your life, and developing your own sensual activities list—and leaving blank lines for add-ons—is what's necessary to keep your sexuality purring above a murmur. New, exotic, and unusual stimuli hold great promise for all of us when it comes to reactivating our sense of feeling powerful, enlivened, and maybe even sexy.

BEING YOUR OWN PLEASURE ACTIVIST

Pleasurable experiences integrated into and interspersed throughout every single day are the key component of preventing or correcting SAS and being a successful pleasure and sexual activist. Variety as the spice of life in combination with a conscious recognition that pleasure is powerful medicine provides an on-ramp to your sexuality by keeping your engine warm and humming.

Deciding what you enjoy and can realistically fit into your life may end up being more difficult than you might expect. In a world so exalting of material consumption, which in turn depends on money and therefore work, finding a balance between work and pleasure is a gargantuan task. If you are a person who grew up in a sensually sterile or atrophic household, trying to decide what is pleasing to you and worth making time for could be hard. There are cultures and families that don't prioritize pleasure and sensuality. People who focus exclusively on being industrious, productive, and accomplished in whatever they take on professionally and personally can have an impossible time wrapping their minds around the value of doing something just because it feels good. Take massage, for example. I have had people say to me, "I don't get it. What's the point of just lying there while someone massages you? I would rather be using the time to take a run and keep up with my daily exercise regimen." Their ambition to achieve things—professional success, monetary wealth, a slim and muscular figure—is what drives their behavior, not their enjoyment of life.

My clients who have lives focused on results and quantifiable data of one sort or another and whose success is determined by measurable productivity don't easily speak the language of sensuality and pleasure. Individuals who work in finance and medicine (especially surgeons), software experts, scientists, statisticians, and engineers—regardless of gender—are often sensually clumsy and naïve. Their acumen for quantitative thinking reflects hardwiring that points them away from sensuality and sensual living, not toward it. Those with an acumen for and a deep appreciation of quantifiable data live almost exclusively in their frontal lobes—where critical thinking and executive processing take place. Frontal lobe thinking isn't bad or naturally exclusive of other types of thought or emotional or physical engagement. But our frontal lobes have their limitations when it comes to the consciousness and appreciation of mind-body pleasures and emotional and intuitive resonance with others. The ability to communicate with other warm-blooded creatures occurs in the midbrain or limbic brain, the epicenter of intuition, feeling, and intimate parlance.

Folks who set up house in their frontal lobes are brainiacs—bright, creative, goal-oriented, and driven individuals who are most comfortable when they can measure their experiences and activities in numbers, graphs, and proportions. This is evidence-based living, and they develop protocols for their behavior from it. Frontal lobe activity and its results are easily quantifiable. Limbic-brain functions are the opposite, and they produce qualitative content, which is often difficult for brainiacs to manage and give full credence to. There is no unit of measurement for intuition, emotion, or pleasure, and therefore, these things are easily rejected by those who look only to what's easily and successfully measurable. This doesn't mean that brainiacs are hopeless or completely disinterested in what goes on in the part of the brain that affects mind-body experiences, like sensuality and sexuality. But they don't tend to have much interest in or fluency with qualitative states. They can also have a high index of suspicion about their *real* value, and they aren't always easy to persuade until push comes to shove and their intimate partners are shouting at the tops of their lungs, "I will leave you if you don't change!"

The daily life of a brainiac is usually filled with all sorts of productive activities. Pleasure for pleasure's sake takes a back seat. A perfect example of this can be found in their commuting practices, especially when they're driving their own cars. A brainiac will listen to the news on the way to and from work, dictate charts, make calls while driving, or attempt to text "important" messages. The idea of listening to a novel or music or simply enjoying the quiet is unnerving to them and can feel like a waste of time. The notion of not being plugged into the world and thinking with a clear result in mind can make them anxious and put them on edge. Changing and expanding these ways of thinking is hard, yet doing so is critically important to improving our relationships to sensual, pleasurable, more powerful living and increasing our access to our sexuality.

So if you are continually adding to your already enormous, dangerously time-consuming workload, incessantly checking e-mails and voice messages, being reticent about turning off your cell phone or e-mail device, and not having rules about eating at a table rather than in your car or somewhere else that will limit your enjoyment of the meal, you may have to work extra hard to live a life of pleasure. If you dislike or dismiss pets as being too much trouble; are always on the go and hesitant to relax and enjoy something like reading, knitting, or listening to music; or live with chronic sleep debt, you really need to consciously choose pleasure, especially if your sex life is less than you and/or your partner want it to be. You must realize that enjoyable activities serve a purpose even if they have no measurable outcome. Grab a novel instead of a newspaper. Stop and notice the aromas of things around you. Be open to trying new flavors, restaurants, and walking paths. Anything that will shake up your senses a bit and wake you up is worth your time and effort. Put aside the goals and competition associated with exercise and just notice how it makes your body feel. And for God's sake, take time off when you get the flu.

To live a fully pleasurable life, we must focus on continually and consciously avoiding repetition of stimuli because it invariably dulls our senses and causes SAS. This is at the root of so many sexual relationships that are well choreographed, scripted, and so predictable we could have sex in our sleep and not wake up. If one or both of you have become like this, it can make for a ticking bomb in the relationship when the other has an awakening that leads to greater awareness about their dissatisfaction. And trust me, this is very likely. One person will experience something that causes them to notice they're starving on the vine—likely in many ways, not just sexually. And this can catapult their partners into feeling resentful of their hunger, even if they too would benefit from an extreme sensual and sexual makeover.

Keeping Sex Alive

There is an element of the sacred in acknowledging that comfort and beauty exist and are there to enjoy. I am not a religious person, but I do identify myself as deeply spiritual and believe the drape between the two is just a gossamer's width. The practices I regularly witnessed my family enjoying left indelible messages about treating life's joys as sacraments as well as the benefit of using pleasure to counterbalance life's woes and heartache. Partaking in something is a way of paying homage, cleansing our souls of sorrow, and expressing gratitude for the jewels available to anyone who pays attention to their presence. Thinking of your pleasure-based practices as tonic for all that ails you will help you stave off SAS and call sexuality into your day-to-day life with greater intention and ease.

The skin-to-skin communion of lovers, the quiet or vociferous intensity of orgasm, and the feelings of being wanted are so indescribably delicious and satisfying that they can be some of life's best medicines. Meaningful sex and self-pleasuring practices can reduce inflammation, ease pain, lessen feelings of isolation, and make you feel that all is right with the world. Pleasure is such a powerful elixir, yet so many of us turn away from it, lose track of its importance in our lives, or disqualify it altogether when it feels inaccessible or effortful. Few of us accept or believe that there's value in cultivating a lifestyle specifically to improve our own sexual experiences and those of our intimate partners without perceiving this as some sort of excessive interest. We are our own saboteurs in our efforts to keep our sexual energy close by.

There was a point in time when colleagues who did not understand my thinking would joke and ask me if sex and pleasure were all I thought about. They also would ask me if I had sex every day. The look of anticipation on their faces was fascinating to me—and bizarre. It felt as though they were baiting me in hopes of learning that my scholarly and personal interests in pleasure and sexuality had a perverse and pathological twist that would reveal itself in my answers to their questions. For those of you reading and waiting for my answer, no, I do not have sex every day; if I did, I would be in an ICU on life support. I am very much the same as many of you reading this book—I am 53, feel brain-dead by 10 P.M., have my own constellation of perimenopausal symptoms that feel decidedly unsexy, and work in a field that can and does interfere with my sexuality when I become entirely too engrossed in it. As for thinking about sex and pleasure all the time, the answer to this is *YES*—and I am proud of it. I am also happy to say that I have come to a place of deep compassion for my clients and myself when we cannot experience pleasure or move into a sexual fantasy, much less have sex, even if our lives depend on it.

As I see it, the primary difference between me and most of the people I counsel is that I see nothing wrong with keeping sex and pleasure in the foreground of my thinking at all times. I have to in order to make my life—and my sexual life—the best they can be. And when this is hard to do, I am willing to examine why, feel sorry for myself, and lick my own paw while thinking, *there, there, dear, you're doing the best you can. Just keep thinking and talking—it will come back eventually.*

My partner and I talk about sex and pleasure in one way or another every day. The conversation between us is ongoing, free associating, and enlivening. We talk about the old days and how frisky we were and admit that we miss those times. We discuss media trends related to sex and my writ-ing—or not writing—about sex. We discuss how to help our patients with sexual problems. We discuss new vibra-tors and the benefits and disadvantages of various brands of lubricants. And we ponder—out loud and to ourselves—the mysterious quality and hold that sex seems to have in so many people's lives. We do our very best to extend this compassion to one another and to ourselves while leading as sensual a life as possible—together as a couple and as individuals. I am convinced that this is what allows us to be as open and comfortable with sex as we are and to stay as sexually active as we do. And even with all that, we too fall off the curb and aren't always as sexually active as we'd like to be or feel is in our best interests. Despite my concerted efforts, I lose track, get distracted, feel exhausted, would rather read a catalog, feel too fat to have sex or too old, or sometimes just can't muster up whatever mysterious thing it is that moves me toward my partner, who I am deeply attracted to and love so much. Welcome to the business of being human, aging, and having baggage, issues, and inexplicable difficulties, just like everyone else.

When we notice that there are too few glossy red hearts on our calendar—our own system for keeping track of when we do have sex—we evaluate the situation and try to figure out what's been keeping us away from something we both dearly love and feel so nourished by. Keeping this going is a lot of work and not always as successful as we want it to be—but it's worth every moment of our time and thought. Even for me, having sex can feel like just one more item on my own to-do list. But the moment I notice this has happened, I pause and deliberately reflect on what has grabbed hold of me and led me astray this time. I am not impervious to life's demands and burdens, a complicated sexual history that can get in the way of pleasure, or the deep, sometimes paralyzing fatigue that can accompany us in life even when we think we're doing all we can to avoid it. This is all the more reason to take frequent advantage of life's pleasures to remind us of how powerful we can feel when we're sensually engaged and how sensuality is just a few steps away from one of the best things life has to offer: sex on our own terms.

QUESTIONS TO ASK YOURSELF

1. Do I do something new that is sensually pleasing every day, and if not, can I make a commitment to do so?

2. What body-based, sensual experiences do I find soothing? Activating? Arousing?

3. What sensually activating things have I considered buying, doing, or seeing, but continue to postpone, and why?

4. What sensually pleasing things could I incorporate into everyday life?

5. Do my partner and I openly talk or write about sex to and with one another with frequency? If not, why? How could we change this?

6. Do I live the life of a brainiac? How can I change this to become more aware of qualitative living and less focused on quantitative living?

7. Am I willing to make the commitment to lead a more sensual life with the intention of being more sexually satisfied? If not, why?

CHAPTER 8

PASSING IT ON

Arriving in the middle of all this, children experience close up and in parallel, often without speaking, all the affections and exiles of their parents' marriage and become not only a close and unconscious student of their relationship, but a sobering mirror of marital happiness and unhappiness from the moment they are toddling around the kitchen, distinguishing right from the scolded wrong. The lessons of marriage are read very early into the textbook of a child's mind.

—DAVID WHYTE

Now that you're at the end of this book, let's go back to the very beginning. The content in the Introduction and Chapter 1 is worth reviewing to get a firm hold on my thesis and to integrate all you've read into your daily lives. Emotional well-being equals powerful living equals increased interest in and access to pleasure of all kinds—including sex. Pleasure begets pleasure, and sexual pleasure is no exception. This is as important to you as an adult woman as it is to the girls in your life whom you love and want the best for.

The markers of emotional well-being—self-esteem, health-seeking behaviors, spiritual satisfaction, resilience, creativity, and compassion—ideally come together and bond to form a necessary and sturdy foundation for developing a healthy relationship with life's pleasures. When they do, a stable, pulsating sexual life develops that can withstand the ardor of normal life and the inevitable storms that affect all long-term relationships. What I have found through my work and my personal life is that an active and satisfying relationship with sex and life's pleasures depends on constant monitoring of the state of our emotional health and its fortitude. This will ultimately shape the expression of our sexuality in relationships more than anything else. There will always be events in life that blow us off course and unseat our markers of emotional wellness, weaken our emotional immunity, and leave us feeling emotionally tattered. But doing the work, no matter how tedious and painful, to mend our psyches after the acute phase of insult has passed has to be an ongoing and conscious choice if what we want is a deep and lasting connection with pleasure, powerful living, and sex.

When I first started working with couples, I believed, as many of my colleagues do, that the etiology of sexual difficulties in couples was directly related to their relational dynamics. Surely, something about how they responded to, reacted to, and interacted with one another was off tempo and the consequence was difficulty with sexual intimacy. This is sometimes true. But it is less often the case when the alchemy of physical attraction has always been present and continues to be, even in the face of decreased sexual desire.

For the longest time, I approached cases of absent libido like a wartime code cracker, determined to uncover the elusive, undercover enemy that was robbing women of their sexual desire. I wanted to discover and reveal what it was about their particular psychology or relationship that had dampened or drained their sexuality to the extent that having sex felt like such a burden. Was I talking with a woman who was concealing an abusive relationship? Was her partner emotionally distant, was she overworked and underappreciated through no fault of her own, or was this a case of a complicated history of sexual abuse that interfered with her owning her sexuality and enjoying it? It wasn't until I started to look at decreased sexual desire as a gender-based issue that I felt better informed about what was happening to so many women who felt sex was effortful, unpleasant, and of no interest to them. The pattern I saw in their lives was a complicated one whose underpinnings were a lack of emotional wellness that left them feeling disempowered and unable to access pleasure in just about anything, and sex was no exception. Identifying this pattern cracked the code, and it is what led me to write this book. I had never read this in anything else on sexuality before; and the more I worked with it, the more I witnessed how it resonated with so many of the women who came to see me for help. This doesn't mean that my work with individuals is formulaic and ignores the particulars of each woman's story. But noting the unequivocal absence of pleasure and sensuality in so many contemporary women's lives has given me a strong foothold for where to start when someone arrives in my office in despair over her lack of interest in sex.

When I first started applying my new theory, I suspected that a lack of time and money would be major contributing factors in lives depleted of pleasure. But as my work progressed with women from all socioeconomic classes, I realized that resources alone won't overpower a mindset that's focused on productivity over pleasure. Women with money, great educations, and free time will crimp and prune their pleasurable interludes just as much as women with far fewer resources. And sensually pleasing living and experiences aren't necessarily dependent on money. The centrifugal force of all women's to-do lists is intense and consistently pulls them away from focusing with intention and a sense of liberation on life's pleasurable pursuits. As some women age and expand their lives to include families and jobs, this can become even more complicated. Faced with the dwindling stamina of age, they toughen their expectations of themselves and work with an outdated reference point for what they *should* be accomplishing in a day. Reports from the front lines of their lives were barren of anything that felt remotely pleasant, with almost every moment of every day consumed by responsibilities and tasks. Pleasure was nowhere in sight.

Many of the women I see are mothers and grandmothers, and sometimes when I am having difficulty convincing a woman that her lifestyle is detrimental to her health, I spin it onto her daughter and ask, "How would you feel if your daughter were living the life you're leading?" This can be very effective in raising their consciousness. When I talk about the impact their lifestyle may be having on the girls they love, some women have no idea how to respond. It has never occurred to them that their sentiments about sex or their paradigm for living is likely to be infecting their daughters in all the wrong ways. Many of us don't realize or choose to forget just how observant and sensitive children are. Girls especially watch their mothers' every move and learn all sorts of things from them about ways to live—or not.

WHAT HAPPENS TO GIRLS

As adults it is our duty not only to give girls an example of a life of regular pleasure seeking, but also to encourage them to tap into their own experiences of pleasure in a healthy way and help them declare how powerful it makes them feel. The assent of women in many professional arenas and academia has resulted in a new generation of girls and women needing to heal their relationships with pleasure and sensuality. We need to define these experiences for ourselves and have the ability to do so when aided by good instruction. When we have daughters who are studious; very attached to academic achievement; and not particularly interested in the arts or physical experiences related to sensual stimuli like clothes, colors, textures, or music, don't revel in relief that she'll somehow be safe in the world because an overt interest in sensuality and sexuality is absent. There needs to be a balance here, and you should strive to help her cultivate her sensual side to guard against the pitfalls of a completely brainiac life.

In contrast, should you see that your young daughter is an especially sensual creature and shows signs of having full-body enjoyment of sensual experiences, don't panic and see this as a very bad sign or a perplexing problem to solve. If your little girl loves wearing twirling skirts and tights without underwear, insists that just the right color and texture of scarf be threaded around her head (or across her groin), tends to want to be naked way past toddlerhood, dances at the age of four *exactly* like Beyoncé, has a perfumer's nose for the most aromatic and expensive body wash, and—oh, worst of all—enjoys masturbating and doesn't work to conceal it, don't assume this means she has a life of sexual promiscuity or stripperdom ahead of her.

Mothers of very sensual little girls arrive in my office dazed, confused, and distraught over their daughters' behaviors. This cohort of little girls shakes the adults around them to the core and leaves them feeling terrified about what they might do next and what might happen when they come of age. The tendency for parents of these kids is to shut them down and quick! Put a stop to that no-underwear business and *absolutely* get them to stop masturbating. It still amazes me that in this advanced day and age, highly intelligent and educated people will ask me with terror, sincerity, and desperation, "What should I do about her masturbating?" And, "Is this normal behavior?" A simple Internet search would answer this question. Yes, it is normal and what to do is simple: Explain to your little girl that touching herself is fine, but she needs to do it in private. (It is worth mentioning here that public masturbation by boys is often treated as a lighthearted matter that's taken in stride—the old "baseball bat" business that many parents and grandparents accept as normal. When I point this out to parents, especially those with boys, they often respond with something like "Well, boys are so like that. And anyway, their penis is on the outside of their body. What else can we expect?" As if that has anything to do with it. The clitoris is also external and feels just as nice when touched as a boy's penis does. In my opinion, public masturbation means touching your genitals for comfort and pleasure in front of people. Boys are not exempt.)

With either boys or girls, open fondling of their genitals in front of people is best managed by not shaming them about it. And with girls especially, we need to use the correct names for anatomy for cryin' out loud! Why do we all call women's genitals en masse a *vagina*? Even *lady parts* would be better—at least that's all-inclusive. This is a golden opportunity for some kick-ass sex education. Nonetheless, euphemisms like *the little man in the boat, your button, cootie-cat, and pousoi* abound. This is not only crazy-town stuff, it also sounds ridiculous coming out of the mouths of smart, contemporary women. It is also an ominous sign of what will happen in the future, when their sensuality-loving girls become slaves to their endocrine systems—and make no mistake about it, this is inevitable.

The squelching of a pleasure-based outlook when our daughters start showing genuine, unstoppable sexiness strikes most of us as the right and responsible thing to do. This is a time when we work our hardest to get them to join a sports team, write for the school newspaper, sing in the choir, or take part in the math club. We're all for anything we think might take their minds off sex. But we forget that the forces of nature will forever be more powerful than we are. While we're screaming *"No!"* and *"Don't you dare!"* their endocrine systems are yelling *"Yes, yes, do!"* Adopting an abstinence-based (or stick-your-head-in-the-sand) model about sex in the hopes that it will distract our girls from sexual feelings and activity will only perpetuate the anesthetized living that this book is trying to help prevent or at least undo. Parenting with an anti-sex attitude will surely lead to SAS. If you believe—as I do—that sensuality can and should help us move toward our sexuality with greater ease, self-confidence, and self-respect, yet you don't want your teen girl to be sexual, then it's likely that you're inadvertently turning her away from both sensuality and sex without even knowing you're doing it. It's a throw-the-baby-out-with-the-bathwater problem.

Giving sexual pleasure a bad reputation means that any affiliated pleasurable activity could be suspect. Better to lose yourself in dieting, academic achievement, and community participation than to pay attention to your pleasure quotient, because it could lead to having sex just for pleasure's sake—perish the thought.

As the mother of a daughter, a midwife for many teens, and the daughter of a mother who was terrified of teen sexuality, I gave this an enormous amount of thought when my own daughter reached early adolescence. I wrote my first book, *The Secret Lives of Teen Girls: What Your Mother Wouldn't Talk about but Your Daughter Needs to Know*, because I knew that being an informed and reliable resource about sex for my daughter was not an aiding-and-abetting felony. The choices she made about sex as a teen were more informed than they would have been if I had pretended she wasn't a beautiful, sexually appealing young woman who generated plenty of interest from others and had sexual interests of her own. I gave thought and consideration to the value of team sports, the school newspaper, and even the math club. But not because I saw them as deterrents to sex, but because I knew they fostered skills that would benefit her in life and help her expand her social and intellectual interests. The two should not be used against one another or thought of as mutually exclusive.

When your daughter or granddaughter turns into a teen, it is positively momentous—and not for all the right reasons. Trust me on this. If you've ever parented a teen girl, you know what I mean. Seemingly from out of nowhere, they transform from a little kid playing with dolls one day to a strange sort of caricature of sexy the next. These are the times when her bulging cleavage makes you want to throw a sweater over her head or her miniskirt is *so* short that all you see is the hemline at the very base of her buttock. Like many unformed beings in the beginning stages of becoming the sophisticated versions of what they actually have in mind, teen girls using their bodies as billboards to announce their sexuality to the world doesn't always come out looking right. This is a hard thing to know how best to react to. What exactly does one say when their teen girl walks into the room looking really stupid but thinking she looks *so hot?* Invariably, your response will be a weird combination of feelings. You'll probably be inclined to laugh or scream in horror, but neither one feels quite right, so what's left?

In order for girls to get the right idea, we need to take a deep breath, stay as calm as possible, move into a soft, wise, and humorous place and say something like "Huh, that's an interesting and different outfit you have on there. It looks like something from *Cake Boss* that didn't come out quite right. How about a little less frosting on the top and more on the base of the cake?" This would be in direct contrast to something like "Jesus *Christ* is the mirror broken in your room? You look like a goddamned whore! Go upstairs this minute and change into something decent!" I highly recommend you choose the first response. You know she'll start to spit nails. But you'll stay calm and she'll reflect on it for a moment (even if it appears otherwise because she winds up not changing anything but her necklace). When you come from this place of compassion and understanding, you'll be more likely to see what is actually happening: this is a girl you love who is trying her sexuality on for size. There is fundamentally nothing wrong with this—no matter how weird or ridiculous she looks. Your mission, should you choose to accept it, is to make your comment and then leave her alone. Caricatures need time to evolve into their real selves, and you just have to be patient. Finesse your guidance with humor and a sureness of knowing that you can spare her from feeling as bad about sex as many women do if you avoid harshly criticizing her awkward experimentation. Pointing her in a different direction without shame, embarrassment, or humiliation for wanting sex in the first place is definitely the way to proceed under these circumstances.

Parenting girls or even being influential family members and friends is a daunting undertaking. At one time in my career as a midwife—because I have been one for so long—the gender of a fetus remained unknown until birth. Many times after a baby was revealed to be a girl, I would hear someone in the labor room say something like "Enjoy her now, because she'll be holy hell later on when she's a teen and you have to keep your eyes on her." For those of us who have spent a lifetime being girls and can read between the lines, the message was clear: Girls are cuter and easier to love when they're little, submissive, asexual, and can't get pregnant, so enjoy this while it lasts. Personally, I am of the reverse mind. It's not that I dislike little girls. But, I really prefer teens, and in part this is because I have such sympathy for how everyone turns against them when they start feeling sexy, being interested in sex, and doing all they can to individuate from their mothers and families. This culture cannot seem to differentiate between a girl who is normally sensual and feels powerful because of it and a girl who is coming on to people indiscriminately and is sexually promiscuous. Any girl who looks or acts sexy is suspected of being a tramp. This deeply saddens me and keeps me very busy as a sexuality counselor. I spend a significant amount of time helping women who were unfortunate enough to have incurred people's wrath and worry over the normal burgeoning of their sexuality during adolescence. Women can reclaim and enjoy their sexuality in adulthood, even when they were forced to conceal or ignore it when it came into their foreground as teens. But it can take time and effort and tremendous support from a safe and encouraging advocate to do this.

The work I do with adult women and teen girls has consistently confirmed what I have personally felt as a woman and what I have observed as a women's health specialist: girls are dissuaded from loving what their bodies can give them—in all sorts of ways. Out of a fear of unplanned pregnancies and STIs, girls are talked out of pursuing things that would be pleasurable by terrified mothers who speak the same shaming vulgarities to their daughters that were flung at them and they have told me were ruinous. It's shame and uncertainty over somatic pleasure that they still carry around like a ball and chain. Mothers who fit the norm will do their best to guide their daughters into a kind of productivity labor camp with academic, professional, and weight-management achievements held on high as the currency for self-esteem, virtuousness, and popularity. Then, 25 (or more) years later I will be listening to their daughters' stories of lost sexual desire and trying to figure out how best to help them relearn—or learn for the first time—how to open the door to pleasure and empowerment through adult sensibilities. With luck and diligence, together, we will successfully unearth her subterranean sexuality.

Adult women have an obligation to little girls, teens, and even older women to take pleasure seriously and utilize it for all it's worth in life. And, don't be afraid of failing at it and feeling as though you have to try and try again. You will, and that is perfectly all right and normal. We are all much more capable of accomplishing many things when we have support, guidance, conviction, and ongoing reminders. We also need to remember that life is full of tumult that has a way of undoing our best and most concerted efforts, and when this happens, we just have to go back to the starting point and begin again. This is true about everything worth doing.

I would never assume that this approach will work for everyone, but if it resonates with you, I suggest the following: write in a journal about how this book made you feel and what it made you think about, make lists of things you really find pleasing, start interjecting things throughout the day that you enjoy and that make you smile, set limits on communicating through technological devices, and go for more face-to-face time with those you love. Buy beautiful stationery and write someone a real letter, walk your dog in a park, listen to music you used to love and something you've never heard before. Try spending an hour a week browsing in a library, choosing a picture book for before-bed reading, going to the movies once a week, eating at a new restaurant, buying something you've never eaten at the grocery store, visiting an old friend you haven't seen in a long time, and making a list of all the places you want to travel to before you die. Keep this book in a place where you'll easily spot it to remind you of pleasure and share it with your beloved and your friends. These are just some ways you can begin to create a life full of pleasure that will lead to feeling more powerful, sensually alive, and, hopefully, sexually energized. We all can do these things—to one extent or another—and they're meaningful things that will give us new ideas, trigger things in ourselves that have been dormant, and introduce us to something new that we might be able to add to our pleasure list.

Make sure to check in with yourself about your markers of emotional well-being often and with rigor. Remind yourself that all kinds of things in life can affect your emotional state and health, and prioritize pleasure as both an ongoing therapy and a curative when things are emotionally trying and sex feels distant. Stop depending on how much you weigh and how much you produce in the world for your self-esteem and start thinking instead about your markers of emotional well-being as the real indicators of wellness and personal success. Do the best you can over and over again, don't give up—no matter how old and dispirited you are—and always remember, I am right in there with you.

ENDNOTES

1. Catherine M. Lynch, "Atropic Vaginitis: Diagnosis and Treatment Option," *The Female Patient,* http://www.femalepatient.com/PDF/035070016.pdf.

2. "What Is a Standard Drink?" National Institute on Alcohol Abuse and Alcoholism, http://www.niaaa.nih.gov/alcohol-health/overview-alcohol-consumption/standard-drink.

3. Eve Ensler, *The Good Body* (New York, Villard, 2004): 5–6.

4. Jonathan Alpert, "In Therapy Forever? Enough Already," *The New York Times,* April 21, 2012, http://www.nytimes.com/2012/04/22/opinion/sunday/in-therapy-forever-enough-already.html.

5. Kate Pickert, "The Man Who Remade Motherhood," *Time,* May 21, 2012, http://www.time.com/time/magazine/article/0,9171,2114427,00.html.

6. Linda Fried in Barbara Strauch, *The Secret Life of the Grown-Up Brain* (New York, Viking, 2010): 49–50.

7. Lynch, "Atropic Vaginitis."

8. To learn more about sex coaching, and Eric, please see http://www.sexlifecoachnyc.com.

9. Louann Brizendine, "Dr. Louann on *Good Morning America* Speaks on *The Male Brain,*" *Good Morning America* video, 3:41, March 24, 2010, http://drlouann.ning.com/video/dr-louann-on-good-morning.

10. Helen Fisher, "8 Surprising Truths About Men," ManoftheHouse.com, May 14, 2011, http://www.equilibrio.com.au/promomail/articles/2012/201202/8_surprising_truths_about_men.html.

BIBLIOGRAPHY

Abraham, Laurie. "What if Our Kids Really Believed We Wanted Them to Have Great Sex?" *The New York Times Magazine,* November 20, 2011.

Ackerman, Diane. *A Natural History of the Senses.* New York: Vintage, 1995.

Alboher, Marci. *One Person, Multiple Careers: A New Model for Work/Life Success.* New York: Warner Business Books, 2007.

Arendash, Gary W. Protecting the Aging Brain: Focus on Nutrition and Mind/Body Health. Institute for Brain Potential—Day-Long Workshop, Tucson, AZ, December, 2011.

Bauer, Carlene. "This Is Your Brain in Love." *Salon.com,* January 27, 2004, http://www.salon.com/2004/01/27/fisher_6/.

Belkin, Lisa. "Keeping Kids Safe from the Wrong Dangers." *The New York Times,* September 19, 2010, New York edition.

Blau, Melinda. "Body Myth." *Mount Holyoke Alumnae Quarterly* (Spring 2011): 8–13.

Bloom, Paul. *How Pleasure Works: The New Science of Why We Like What We Like.* New York: W. W. Norton & Company, 2010.

Brisendine, Louann. *The Female Brain.* New York: Three Rivers Press, 2006.

———. *The Male Brain: A Breakthrough Understanding of How Men and Boys Think.* New York: Three Rivers Press, 2010.

Bureau of Labor Statistics. The Editor's Desk. "Labor Force Participation of Women and Mothers, 2008." October 9, 2009, http://www.bls.gov/opub/ted/2009/ted_20091009.htm.

Burrows, L.J. and Kimberly Resnick-Anderson. "Female Orgasmic Disorder." *The Female Patient* 36, no. 6 (June 2011): 18–21.

Castleman, Michael. "Desire in Women: Does it Lead to Sex? Or Result from It?" *Psychology Today* (July 15, 2009): www.psychologytoday.com/node/30942.

Chollet, Janet A. "Progress in Vulvovaginal Atrophy Treatment." *The Female Patient* 35 (December 2010): 29–31.

Dowd, Maureen. *Are Men Necessary?: When Sexes Collide.* New York: Penguin Audio, 2005.

Fast, Julius. *The Pleasure Book.* New York: Stein and Day, 1975.

Gawande, Atul. Annals of Medicine. "Letting Go." *The New Yorker* (August 2, 2010): www.newyorker.com/reporting/2010/08/02/100802fa_fact_gawande.

Gore, Ariel. *Bluebird: Women and the New Psychology of Happiness.* New York: Farrar, Straus, and Giroux, 2010.

Gorney, Cynthia. "The Estrogen Dilemma." *The New York Times,* April 14, 2010, http://www.nytimes.com/2010/04/18/magazine/18estrogen-t.html?adxnnl=1&adxnnlx=131&_r=1.

Gottman, John and Nan Silver. *The Seven Principles for Making Marriage Work: A Practical Guide from the Country's Foremost Relationship Expert.* New York: Three Rivers Press, 1999.

Groopman, Jerome. Books. "God on the Brain." *The New Yorker* (September 17, 2001): www.newyorker.com/archive/2001/09/17/010917crbo_books.

Gross, Jane. "A Doctor's Undivided Focus on the Minds of the Elderly." *The New York Times,* May 1, 2011, New York edition.

Hinchliff, Sharron and Merryn Gott. "Seeking Medical Help for Sexual Concerns in Mid- and Later Life: A Review of the Literature," *Journal of Sex Research* 48, nos. 2–3 (March 2011): 106–117.

Iacono, Valeria Lo. "10 Famous Belly Dancers," *World Belly Dance:* www.worldbellydance.com/Top-10/10-famous-belly-dancers.html.

International Longevity Center. *Intimacy and Sexuality: Toward a Lifespan Perspective.* New York: International Longevity Center-USA, 2006.

Katz, Anne. *Breaking the Silence on Cancer and Sexuality: A Handbook for Healthcare Providers.* Pittsburgh: Oncology Nursing Society, 2007.

Kinsley, Craig H. and Elizabeth Meyer. "Maternal Mentality." *Scientific American Mind* (July/August 2011): 25–30.

Krychman, Michael. "Impact of Vaginal Atrophy of Quality of Life and Sexuality." *OBG Management* 22, no. 11 (November 2010): http://www.obgmanagement.com/article_pages.asp?AID=9285.

LaFraniere, Sharon. "For Many Chinese, New Wealth and a Fresh Face." *The New York Times,* April 24, 2011, New York edition.

Lehrer, Jonah. *How We Decide.* Boston, New York, NY: Houghton Mifflin Harcourt, 2009.

Linden, David J. *The Compass of Pleasure: How Our Brains Make Fatty Foods, Orgasm, Exercise, Marijuana, Generosity, Vodka, Learning, and Gambling Feel So Good.* New York: Viking, 2011.

Love, Susan M. and Alice D. Domar. *Live a Little!: Breaking the Rules Won't Break Your Health.* New York: Crown Archetype, 2009.

Madsen, Pamela. *Shameless: How I Ditched the Diet, Got Naked, Found True Pleasure…and Somehow Got Home in Time to Cook Dinner.* New York: Roadale, 2011.

McCarthy, Barry. Restoring and Revitalizing Marital Sexuality. Health Education Network—Workshop. Grand Rapids, Michigan. October 2011.

Mead, Rebecca. Gender Studies. "The End?" *The New Yorker,* October 10, 2011, pp. 36–38.

Melby, Todd. "In the Mood: The Intersection of Negative Mood and Sexuality." *Contemporary Sexuality* 45, no. 6 (June 2011): 1, 4-5.

Moalem, Sharon. *How Sex Works: Why We Look, Smell, Taste, Feel, and Act the Way We Do.* New York: HarperCollins, 2009.

"Mommy's Helper, in Red and White, and in the Courtroom, Too." *The New York Times,* April 24, 2011, New York edition.

National Institute on Alcohol Abuse and Alcoholism: www.niaaa.nih.gov.

Paul, Pamela. "When Thoughts Turn to Sex, or Not." *The New York Times,* December 11, 2011, New York edition.

Resh, Evelyn. *The Secret Lives of Teen Girls: What Your Mother Wouldn't Talk about but Your Daughter Needs to Know.* Carlsbad, California: Hay House, 2009.

Roberts, Jeff. "Wine for 'Mommy' Sets Off Trademark Fight," *Reuters,* April 20, 2011, www.reuters.com/article/2011/04/21/us-wine-mommy-idUSTRE73K.

Rosenbloom, Stephanie. "Ambition + Desire = Trouble." *The New York Times,* June 19, 2011, New York edition.

Rothschild, Babette. *The Body Remembers: The Psychophysiology of Trauma and Trauma Treatment.* Boston: W. W. Norton & Company, Incorporated, 2000.

Rozhon, Tracie, "To Have, Hold and Cherish, Until Bedtime," *The New York Times,* March 11, 2007, http://www.nytimes.com/2007/03/11/us/11separate.html?pagewanted=all.

Rubin, Gretchen. *The Happiness Project: Or, Why I Spent a Year Trying to Sing in the Morning, Clean My Closets, Fight Right, Read Aristotle, and Generally Have More Fun.* New York: Harper, 2009.

Schalet, Amy. "Must We Fear Adolescent Sexuality?" *Medscape General Medicine* 6, no. 4 (2004): 44.

Strauch, Barbara. *The Secret Life of the Grown-Up Brain: The Surprising Talents of the Middle-Aged Mind.* New York: Viking Adult, 2010.

Strom, Stephanie. "A City Tries to Slim Down." *The New York Times,* June 14, 2011, New York edition.

Sulak, Patricia J. "Critique Your Caloric Consumption." *The Female Patient* 36 (December 2011): 14–19.

Thurber, James and E.B. White. *Is Sex Necessary?: Or Why You Feel the Way You Do.* New York: Harper Brothers, 1929.

Tiefer, Leonore: www.leonoretiefer.com.

Townsend, Angela. "University Hospitals Program Treating Women's Sexual Dysfunction." *Cleveland.com,* June 4, 2012, http://www.cleveland.com/healthfit/index.ssf/2012/06/uh_is_the_latest_cleveland-are.html.

Tulley, Gever. "5 Dangerous Things you Should Let Your Kids Do: Gever-Tully on Ted.com." TED University 2007, pre-conference program, http://blog.ted.com/2007/12/21/gever_tulley_on/.

"Untangling the Web of Low Desire." *Contemporary Sexuality* 43, no. 11 (November 2009): 1, 3–5.

U.S. Department of Health and Human Services, National Institute on Alcohol Abuse and Alcoholism. "Alcohol: A Woman's Health Issue." NIH Publication No. 03 4956, Revised 2008, http://pubs.niaaa.nih.gov/publications/brochurewomen/women.htm.

"US Low Score on World Motherhood Rankings: Charity." *AFP Global Edition,* May 4, 2010, http://www.thefreelibrary.com/US+low+score+on+world+motherhood+rankings%3a+charity-a01612210249.

Webber, Rebecca. "Are You With the Right Mate?" *Psychology Today* (January/February 2012): 59–64.

Weekes, Karen. *Women Know Everything: 3,241 Quips, Quotes & Brilliant Remarks.* Philadelphia: Quirk Books, 2007.

Weiner, Ellis. Shouts & Murmurs. "Just in Time for Spring." *The New Yorker,* March 28, 2011, p. 59.

Whyte, David. *The Three Marriages: Reimagining Work, Self and Relationship.* New York: Riverhead Books, 2009.

Williams, Alex. "Quality Time, Redefined." *The New York Times,* May 1, 2011, New York edition.

Wolfe, Alexandra. What Were They Thinking? "A Purity Ball, Oroville, Calif." *The New York Times Sunday Magazine,* November 13, 2011.

Zoldbrod, Aline. Assessing Intrapsychic Blocks to Sexual Pleasure Using the Milestones of Sexual Development Model. *Contemporary Sexuality* 37, no. 11 (November 2003): 7–13.

ACKNOWLEDGMENTS

I am a solitary writer. In order for me to concentrate on my work and do my best, I have to be isolated, write in the morning, and keep my ideas mostly to myself. That's all the more reason I need the best editor possible, an editor who knows my voice, style, and content, and who also really knows how to critique nonfiction.

Working with Laura Gray at Hay House Publishers is one of the top ten great things that has ever happened to me. She inherited me from Patty Gift, who remains in the background, ever present, and who fortified my self-confidence and writing style by working with me on my first book. At that time, Laura was not the boss of me. This time around, I am all hers, and I couldn't be happier. She has extraordinary editing talents, and we share an appreciation for humor that's just so right. Saying thank you will never be enough. Sally Mason, a careful and voluminous reader, helped Laura in her editing efforts. Thanks, Sally. I could feel you in the background.

My agent also inherited me. Jennifer Weltz was appointed the task of managing me by her mother, Jean Naggar, who, like Patty Gift, passed me along knowing that I would always do my best and with an eye for a great match. Jennifer is fantastic! She is smart, capable, and as close to perfect as I could imagine an agent being. Thank you, Jean and Jennifer, for representing me in the United States and abroad and for your incomparable support, critical feedback, and superb way of allowing me to be myself while preventing me from getting in my own way.

There are people who have helped me formulate and fine-tune my ideas and paradigm and who aren't ever afraid to tell me I am wrong about something or fill me in on thoughts and feelings of their own about sex, power, and pleasure. They have also supported my work in countless ways, directly and indirectly: Max Rivinus, Howard Schultz, Andrew Wolf, Cary Barbor-Zahaby, Dianne Dunkelman, Gayle Kabaker, Cindy Geyer, Mark Liponis, Carolanne McKirnan, Larry Gold, Corissa Gold, and all the organizers of the Conference on World Affairs, CUBoulder. A special thanks to Paula Zoito, Paula Paradise, Melissa Wood, Rachelle Bleau, Shari Cristofolini, Erin Lawson, Karen Shoestock, Sara Sawyer, Susan Yates, Chuck O'Neill, and Alison Hastings—all of whom have been tirelessly interested and supportive of my work and filled my life with learning, laughter, and comfort; I love working with all of you.

My mother, sister, and aunt don't really understand what I do, but they support me anyway. Thanks for this and for the ways you have influenced my writing and perspective on what's most important in life. Your love for and support of the arts have been an important influence all my life. My sister once told me that she loved being Greek so much that if she could, she would wear an Evzone's uniform every day. While I wouldn't go that far, I do understand and share some of the underpinnings of her sentiment.

I have had the extraordinary good fortune to have Mark Immerman as my friend for more than 30 years. He never has a harsh word for me and laughs at all my jokes, even when the situation at hand is grim. We keep one another buoyant and flexible and attached to life in many ways, even under very difficult circumstances. Everyone should be as lucky as I am to have someone like him as their friend. His beautiful smile and appreciation for life and all its pleasures—big and small—inspire me personally and have deeply influenced my writing and my belief that laughing at things, even when they're not funny, makes all the difference in living life to its fullest or not.

Since the age of 12, my friend Matthew Hock has been patient, open, and supportive of me in all my endeavors. He has a great way of encapsulating a meaningful thought with fabulous brevity. We talk about everything, including sex, without rules or limits on the conversation. His voice and steadfast friendship have been medicine for me for over 40 years. I love him dearly and feel loved back.

John Miner, M.D., worked with me on this project, my first book, and countless other things for 18 years. His varied contributions to my work and personal life have made much of what I do and experience possible. Our frequent and regular contact had to end in 2011 but that doesn't really matter. This is one of those situations in life when I'm reminded of how our definition and concepts of time, space, and the present can't and don't apply. His influence is everlasting. There isn't a day that goes by that I don't think of him, thank him, and wish him nothing but the best that life has to offer.

Charlie Swenson is someone I am just getting to know, and so far I love what I see. He is one of the most attentive listeners I have ever had a conversation with and his feedback has proven valuable, insightful, and comforting. He came into my work on this book toward the end of my writing, but he helped in significant ways, nonetheless. I have to thank him for his quick and accurate read of what I needed most and for keeping up with my pace.

My daughter is in a category of influence all her own. Thalia lives a life so influenced by pleasure and the power it grants her that I can't help but learn from her on a regular basis. Despite being in her early 20s, she is a sophisticated sensualist who has found a place to be that speaks to her zest for life and love of earthly delights. She is a great teacher, and I hope that my perspective on life has helped point her in the direction she's gone in, even though it's taken her miles away. She's a beauty, in so many ways.

At the end of so many authors' acknowledgments pages is a tribute to their spouse. Many folks give thanks for their partner's support because they left them alone to write, took care of kids, cleaned the house, or read their manuscripts over and over again. Some of these things are true about my spouse, Robin. But, what's most important is that she stands next to me, day in and day out, with the same desire and intention to keep pleasure, power, and sex alive and well. Our relationship has informed my work, strengthened my commitment to living joyously, and forced me to be true to my word; I have lucked out in this life beyond my wildest dreams.

ABOUT THE AUTHOR

Evelyn Resh, MPH, CNM, is a certified sexuality counselor with the American Association of Sexuality Educators, Counselors and Therapists. She is also a certified nurse-midwife and has been in practice for more than 20 years. Resh holds a master of public health degree and undergraduate degrees in nursing, psychology, and medical anthropology. She draws from her experience as a midwife and sexuality counselor in her integrative approach to women's health. Resh lectures frequently across the country to professional and lay audiences on the topics of women's health and sexual satisfaction. She is especially known for her warm, lively, and good-humored approach to her subject matter and her ability to make others feel comfortable with hard-to-discuss topics.

Website: www.evelynresh.com

Hay House Titles of Related Interest

YOU CAN HEAL YOUR LIFE, the movie,
starring Louise L. Hay & Friends
(available as a 1-DVD program and an expanded 2-DVD set)
Watch the trailer at: **www.LouiseHayMovie.com**

THE SHIFT, the movie,
starring Dr. Wayne W. Dyer
(available as a 1-DVD program and an expanded 2-DVD set)
Watch the trailer at: **www.DyerMovie.com**

♂♀

*ARE YOU TIRED AND WIRED?: Your Proven 30-Day Program
for Overcoming Adrenal Fatigue and Feeling Fantastic,*
by Marcelle Pick, MSN, OB/GYN NP

ECSTASY IS NECESSARY: A Practical Guide, by Barbara Carrellas

THE FATIGUE SOLUTION: Increase Your Energy in Eight Easy Steps,
by Eva Cwynar, M.D.

*GREAT SEX, NATURALLY: Every Woman's Guide to Enhancing
Her Sexuality Through the Secrets of Natural Medicine,*
by Dr. Laurie Steelsmith and Alex Steelsmith

All of the above are available at your local bookstore,
or may be ordered by contacting Hay House (see next page).

♂♀

We hope you enjoyed this Hay House book. If you'd like
to receive our online catalog featuring additional information
on Hay House books and products, or if you'd like
to find out more about the Hay Foundation, please contact:

Hay House, Inc., P.O. Box 5100, Carlsbad, CA 92018-5100
(760) 431-7695 or (800) 654-5126
(760) 431-6948 (fax) or (800) 650-5115 (fax)
www.hayhouse.com® • **www.hayfoundation.org**

ॐ

Published and distributed in Australia by:
Hay House Australia Pty. Ltd., 18/36 Ralph St., Alexandria NSW 2015
Phone: 612-9669-4299 • *Fax:* 612-9669-4144 • www.hayhouse.com.au

Published and distributed in the United Kingdom by:
Hay House UK, Ltd., 292B Kensal Rd., London W10 5BE • *Phone:*
44-20-8962-1230 • *Fax:* 44-20-8962-1239 • www.hayhouse.co.uk

Published and distributed in the Republic of South Africa by:
Hay House SA (Pty), Ltd., P.O. Box 990, Witkoppen 2068
Phone/Fax: 27-11-467-8904 • www.hayhouse.co.za

Published in India by: Hay House Publishers India, Muskaan Complex,
Plot No. 3, B-2, Vasant Kunj, New Delhi 110 070*Phone:*
91-11-4176-1620 • *Fax:* 91-11-4176-1630 • www.hayhouse.co.in

Distributed in Canada by: Raincoast, 9050 Shaughnessy St.,
Vancouver, B.C. V6P 6E5 • *Phone:* (604) 323-7100
Fax: (604) 323-2600 • www.raincoast.com

ॐ

Take Your Soul on a Vacation

Visit **www.HealYourLife.com®** to regroup, recharge,
and reconnect with your own magnificence.
Featuring blogs, mind-body-spirit news, and life-changing
wisdom from Louise Hay and friends.

Visit **www.HealYourLife.com** today!

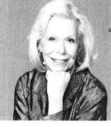

Lightning Source UK Ltd.
Milton Keynes UK
UKOW040228050413

208708UK00001B/15/P